Prancercise®:

The Art of Physical and Spiritual Excellence

By

Joanna Rohrback

Preface by Internationally renowned Dr. E.K.Schandl

WingSpan Press

With special thanks to Eric Gzimalowski for the cover and to Karen J. Hatzigeorgiou of Karenswhimsy.com, for access to illustrations

Printed in the United States of America
Published by WingSpan Press, Livermore, CA
www.wingspanpress.com
The WingSpan name, logo and colophon
are the trademarks of WingSpan Publishing.

Publisher's Cataloging-in-Publication Data

Rohrback, Joanna.
Prancercise : the art of physical and spiritual excellence / by Joanna Rohrback ; preface by internationally renowned E.K.Schandl.
p. cm.
ISBN 978-1-59594-480-1 (pbk.)
ISBN 978-1-59594-690-4 (hardcover)
ISBN 978-1-59594-793-2 (ebk.)
1. Aerobic exercises. 2. Physical fitness. 3. Exercise.   I. Schandl, E.K. II. Title.
RA781.15 .R64 2012
613.7—dc23
2012948261

DISCLAIMER: The protocols or health recommendations in this book are solely the testimonial of the author as to what she has practiced successfully for herself and intends this book to be for educational purposes alone and not medical advice. If you deem it necessary please seek the advice of a medical professional

THIS BOOK IS DEDICATED TO MY DECEASED FATHER WHOSE RELENTLESS CONFIDENCE IN ME HAS COMPELLED ME TO FOLLOW MY DREAMS…

AND TO ALL THE" FREE THINKERS" OF THE WORLD, MAY THEY TOO REALIZE THEIRS…

PREFACE

"Prancercise® by Joanna Rohrback is a delightful study and instructions of physical and spiritual freedom created by movement. The idea goes back as far as 1600A.D. The practitioner takes time to focus away from the world around him and concentrates more on knowing and expressing himself in terms of the world outside. Prancercise® is a dynamic form of dance, created by the dancer, that enhances breathing, muscle strength, coordination, endurance and spiritual fulfillment. Combined with music, it may be an individually constructed work of performing arts."

Dr. E. K. Schandl Clinical Biochemist, Oncobiologist

MS; PHD; FACB; CC(NRCC); SC(ASCP); LNC

http://americanmetaboliclaboratories.net/Dr._Schandl_C.html

TABLE OF CONTENTS

INTRODUCTION

Prancercise® may be considered a revolutionary form of aerobics someday. Just as Isadora Duncan revolutionized dance with her new techniques and approaches at the turn of the century, so do I project Prancercise® could change the course of approaches and techniques towards fitness indefinitely. Actually Isadora changed more than dance in and of itself; she spurred a change in the attitudes and social mores of her time as well as those of the approaching eras. I suspect so too could Prancercise®.

Prancercise® is meditative yet, it is far removed from yoga. It incorporates rhythmic movement in it, yet it is far removed from aerobic dance and Jazzercise, which are both regimented. In contrasting Prancercise® with other existing exercise programs, I will parallel it to the movement of horses, analyzing this inherent characteristic of the exercise (form of movement). Isn't this lean muscular creature of strength and endurance, the horse, a better model for us to seek in fitness than a superficial steroid king or queen on the cover of a magazine?

In the execution of a Prancercise® program you'll incorporate music to induce movement however, the music used is preferably not a standardized composite like that which is used in a typical health club class or on an aerobics video. After a Prancercise® session you shouldn't feel as though you "worked out;" you should rather feel like you played for a while like jumping over the waves at the beach. You should not only feel more relaxed, but even up lifted, since you nurture your spirit with this unique exercise. Yes, we can almost regain our youth through this marvelous exercise. It instills the child like qualities in us that have been buried under layers of negative social conditioning. After prancercising regularly you may notice greater self-confidence, as the exercise reinforces your self-identity and individuality, lending itself to a feeling of thankfulness that you are you!

Aren't most of us getting lost in the multitudes these days? Should we be striving to all look like top paid models or actors? Should our behavior be predictable like that of a popular character on a T.V. show, or a computer program? Do we really want to be clones of what society sells us as desirable? We could strive to become like a Farrah Faucett automaton; however, don't we really need and prefer to be ourselves? Yes, it was my rising need to be and express myself as an individual that lent itself to the birth of this unique exercise. It's the only child I ever expect to bear!

In consideration of the intellectual potential of this program, I will present to the reader a variety of methods that he or she could employ to develop greater self-awareness and a higher state of consciousness.

Through avenues of meditation and forms of detachment, and in implementing one's own inner rhythm as well as other sounds, we can gain more insight into ourselves and achieve more from the program.

.

Through adhering rigidly to my definitive beliefs and principles, I've been able to derive a great degree of interrelationship between my program and many higher principles of living, in accordance with natural law. Many of these higher principles were reinforced by the Classic Greek and Roman philosophers, which I attempt to integrate into this book. By including a chapter on injury prevention, I hope to offer the reader that extra measure of consideration that will facilitate a more pleasurable personal experience, if he or she attempts a Prancercise® program for themselves. I offer a basic format of the anatomy and physiology inherent in the execution of this form of exercise. Why are we continuing to beat our bones in sports like running and racquet ball or a profession and hobby like ballet?

In the same light, I wish to present what I consider the most favorable dietary guidelines that will complement a Prancercise® program. By highlighting the merit and common sense of "Diet for a New America" by John Robbins, the principles of Mahatma Gandhi, and the underlying dietary considerations of vegetarianism, of which the horse is certainly a disciple; I hope to achieve this objective. I wish to awaken a serious interest in the reader of the value that a vegetarian diet can be to the person desiring to achieve the ultimate in fitness and the highest ideals by which to live.

Through the synthesis of the knowledge presented in this literary resource, one could conceivably bring them self to question what kind of imaginary country could exist, if everyone living there adhered to the principles presented in this work. This is why I've concluded my book by illustrating my vision of a Utopian society. By doing this I hope to have laid the foundation for many questions concerning our current manner of existence. Socrates, around 330 B.C. in his rhetorical manner took a similar approach, as he instigated people to question their existence. In my speculative premise I will suggest how an alternate social order of existence could lend itself to a more peaceful and loving world. Prancercise® can be a vehicle to quash any violent tendencies you might possess. It can induce greater animation, vitality and constructiveness in your existence; replacing violent and emotionless behavior. Why don't we exercise outdoors and take a bath in nature, so necessary for physical and mental well being? If our current rate of planetary destruction continues, we soon won't have the choice. We may see the day there are no trees and wildlife to inspire us while we exercise. We may be forced to exercise indefinitely in superficial, unnatural surroundings that are boring and emotionally cold. After all, as Chief Seattle a great American Indian stated: "All things are connected."

If indeed, every breath we take, every step we execute, and every word we choose to speak, somehow affects all that's around us; should we not consider the intrinsic and extrinsic value of all our actions, and live in greater harmony with each other and the planet? It is from this perspective, and with these notions in mind, that I'm attempting to present my Prancercise® program.

"A happy life is one which is in accordance with its own nature."

—Seneca

"If a man doesn't keep pace with his companions, perhaps it is because he hears a different drummer. Let him keep step to music which he hears, however measured or far away."

—Henry David Thoreau

"My life is for itself and not for a spectacle… what I must do is all that concerns me, not what the people think."

—Ralph Waldo Emerson

"Whatever you do may seem insignificant, but it is most important that you do it."

—Mahatma Gandhi

CHAPTER ONE

Prancercise®: The Definition, Mechanics, and Evolution of it

It all started back in 1989, what seems like a century has passed since then... I started writing about this new form of aerobics I had developed, and my life at this time. I wrote of why this exercise was not a contrived development, but a very natural occurrence. Yes, it was actually back in the beginning of 1989, that I sat down in my papason chair to commence upon the most exciting project of my entire life, up to this point. It was but three months earlier that I had broken off my engagement to marry a handsome and charming Jewish Dentist, two years my junior. Although he loved me very much, I knew in my heart that our objectives were all too disparate. I knew I was never meant to assume a traditional lifestyle. The nearer we came to considering a wedding date and the more I found myself in a traditional role, the more miserable I became. I was inundated with grocery shopping, ironing and the planning of weekend social activities. Each boring day led to another boring week and month, fighting to maintain a spark of autonomy. I found it increasingly difficult to continue maintaining my dietary and fitness habits. My dietary habits were based on wholesome natural foods, high in fiber, low in calories. Although I kept such foods available in the apartment, I was forced to overlook Entenman's pound cake and Breyer's ice cream to get to them.

Since I worked fewer hours than my boyfriend, earning considerably less than he, my responsibilities as a house servant were expected more than appreciated. With every passing day my self-esteem plummeted. I dreaded the weekends worst of all because it usually meant going to a boring movie or overindulging in even more sinful food at a restaurant.

I began to realize more and more each day, how my values and lifestyle really conflicted with those of my future husband's. Regardless, it was primarily the requirement to have a child that was the icing on the cake for me. I had struggled with this notion since I was young child myself.

As I aged my mother was especially good at making me feel "desperate" for security and a family. Never a thought was given to fulfilling my creative desires, which were forever on hold. I realized if I was to have a child at age 36 or thereafter, there was an increasing chance it wouldn't be normal. Additionally, I would probably lose my hard earned shape and even more of the freedom I needed to fulfill my creative desire (which was more aesthetic than physical). Here I had only just started battling for creative "time out" from the mainstream, and I was losing it. With the pressing added responsibilities of marriage and a child, I saw all too clearly the writing on the wall.

After two weeks of grieving I left my fiancé and moved into my own apartment. How excited I was, since there were only two other brief instances where I had actually lived alone, no roommates or family. I had been so happy at those times. I moved about one hundred boxes myself, working day and night for about a week. I also arranged for some basic upgrades, such as a new air conditioning unit and new carpet. I made a cute and peaceful sanctuary out of a rather neglected little beach studio. It was fortunate that my new home was in a prime location, only about a mile up the beach from where I had resided with my fiancé. My new apartment was even closer to a strip of the beach called the "Broadwalk," in Hollywood, Florida. This section of the beach was a haven for exercise fanatics, like myself; so sets the stage for the creation of prancercising.

You will best comprehend the evolution of this unique exercise, by being briefed a little further on my background and personality. As I mentioned earlier, I'm very non-traditional in every sense of the word. As a child, I forever sought out mischief. I suspect that the excitement and intrigue I derived from it, gave me an endless means of entertainment. I found it a necessity to break the boredom of growing up like an only child. My sisters well my seniors, were both in college when I was six. In addition to mischief, music and dancing were favorite pastimes of mine. One of the first sizeable gifts my father graced me with was a child's phonograph. I was about three or four years old when I received this most prized possession. Every night thereafter, my father would arrive home from his long commute to work, with another new record for me. It was the fifties and hits like "The Green Door" were popular. I would dance tirelessly to music from my records, the radio, or just some songs I knew and sang. Whenever my parents had company, I found an instant audience. I always took full advantage of these opportunities to be a star. I later came to realize that dancing and music were two of my favorite escapes from the horrors of the household I grew up in.

My parents fought ceaselessly. My mother further compounded my uneasiness, by letting me know I was no "wanted" child. She never hesitated to enlighten me with the fact that my conception was the result of my father's rape of her. Now you must understand my father was as nonviolent as a lamb, so rape, in my mother's eyes was simply not preferring to have sex, when having it. It's likely that my mother figured she was raped on a regular occasion, since she never had a favorable thing to say concerning sex her entire life. My poor father poured all the love he was deprived of sharing with my mother into me. Needless to say, this really fueled a fire in her towards me. She managed to express her frustration, by allotting me with regular beatings and harsh, cruel words that were demeaning and defacing. My father would come home, weak and tired from his day's tribulations at work, only to have her anxiously attack him, with long explanations of my demon-like disobedience. "She can't be controlled" and " she's no damn good," she would scowl. Consequently, it was not uncommon to receive a final lashing from him. My father would usually come to his senses, finally, and fervently apologize to me. I never however, felt I needed to forgive him since I understood the reasons for his behavior. It was always very clear to me that my father loved me sincerely and unconditionally. It was this love and this love alone, that nurtured whatever good was to ever come from me. By the time I reached eight years old, my father started sending me to camp for the summers. He would let me select the camps that advertised the most elite amenities. My paramount concern was the quality and quantity of the camp's horseback riding, pet care and dancing programs. My first experience away was most exciting. I attended a camp in the Berkshires that had an excellent dance department. I can recall signing up to try out for the exclusive dance play that the department held near the end of the summer. This would be viewed by the camper's families as well as local residents of the area. Most of the summer was spent in preparation for this production. There I was, a homely looking girl, short, curly, frizzy, brown hair, a bit of a belly and a larger than average size nose. Furthermore, I hadn't had a single dance lesson under my belt! Then there were the others… pretty pink tutus and leotards, blonde little ponytails bobbing behind cute little tushies. Why they'd been told they were little ballerinas ever since they could remember…Well the teachers called upon us one at a time, to present ourselves atop a huge stage. We were to dance to this one particular piece of Jazz, totally unrehearsed so I observed those rehearsing ahead of me very carefully, embracing a clever move or two. However, my most vivid memory is of how very much I wanted a part and how much I loved to dance. Upon my turn to rehearse, I climbed up on the stage, closed my eyes, and felt the music deep down to the core of my existence. After about a minute or two of watching me move, the director exclaimed "that's enough, we've got our lead" and hence I was chosen for it.

I played the part of "Madeline" in the story about a sickly little thing of a girl, at a strict Catholic girls' school. I danced in all the dance routines and in addition had a scene or two to dance solo. In these solo scenes I was given full improvisational rights. This all was like a dream, I was in heaven.

By the age of ten I was directing musicals for my neighborhood. I would cast the neighborhood children into various roles. They would then sing and dance to plays I created and directed. Yes, entertaining, dance and music sparked a fire in me. My favorite television shows were naturally old musicals. Some of my very favorites were the Fred Astaire/Ginger Rogers movies. I also cherished all of the Judy Garland and Gene Kelly pictures.

When my adolescence arrived, somehow life seemed to go from the Emerald City and the Wizard of Oz to Heartbreak Hotel. I was haunted by one empty love affair after another. My experiences seemed to be reflections of the unfulfilled desires and unhappiness my parents faced. It appears it wasn't until I began my work with Prancercise® that the independence and peace I sought all those past years came trickling into my life. I had finally found my most perfect natural and instinctive outlet for the accumulating frustrations which stemmed from numerous empty male/female relationships. Through a better understanding of my real needs and having some healthy outlets for them, I was able to slowly reconstruct the purpose of my existence. Inherent in fulfilling this purpose, was seeking to gain harmony, peace and balance in my life. This inevitably would require balancing myself; emotionally, intellectually and physically.

Prancercise® became concrete approximately one month after I had separated from my fiancé I had adopted an exceptionally rigid and extensive exercise program. I was determined to once again attempt to rid my thighs of the cellulite they were adorned with since a very early age. I included in my program of cross conditioning a composite of stretching, biking, power walking, and running. Spiritually I was exceptionally happy these days. Promptly after my last relationship with the Dentist, another man entered my life. He had nearly an identical belief system to my own, or so I dreamily convinced myself. At the height of this short lived interlude, I found myself very intoxicated with life. One morning while in my usual high spirits, while power walking, with ankle weights on, there must of been an exceptionally good song on my Walkman, cause as I attempted to stretch my legs to get the maximum muscle tone in my buttocks, hips and thighs, I somehow started naturally rocking and twisting my whole body. As I proceeded, my arms started following the rest of my body, in rhythm. The next thing I knew, I was nearly dancing, but not quite. I hadn't given way from a strong stretching stride; it was really quite amazing. Needless to say, I was an eyesore. My normal walk had always been quite girlish, more of a wiggle than a walk. Now this exaggerated wiggle, speeded up and stretched out with arms moving in harmony, was the beginnings of Prancercising. Now at the conclusion of my power walking session of twenty five minutes, I was accustomed to running back to my point of origin so consequently, when it was time to come back, I experienced another amazing occurrence. I now removed the ankle weights and placed them around my wrists, considering upper body development and the need to reduce knee strain caused from running with them on my ankles. So now at a quickened pace, with the ankle weights on my wrists, I was doing a combination of shadow boxing, running and prancing.... At times I looked very similar to a boxer in the ring, yet other times when I'd leap into the air, more like an antelope. If you could imagine these images with continued movement forward, incorporating a type of two steps or rocking sideways, you could conceive of another variation of this aerobics. Yes my life had changed forever, Prancercise® was definitely born. I venture to doubt that a mother delivering a healthy baby for the first time, could not have been prouder or more fulfilled than I did the moment Prancercise® was born. Very much like a newborn being nurtured, Prancercise® grew and developed day by day. New steps and movements took shape naturally, especially as new music was incorporated into my routine.

Before I knew it, the days of using my new program, turned into months. My staying power with my new program was no surprise to me. One reason for this was because it afforded me an integration of body and soul in a non competitive manner. The time it took, the intensity of movement during that time and the distance covered were not considerations to me, like it might be for most power walkers or runners. For me this was no work out, it was more a form of psychotherapy. I found the more I prancercised, the more I was becoming in touch with my true identity. Dance, which Prancercise® is a variation of, is a fine natural form of self-expression. It goes much further than being just a mere outlet for stress; it requires a defined expression of one's emotions through movement. If you are happy, angry or even depressed it can all be reflected through your movement. Consequently, your spectators are being communicated with though not too directly or personally. The advantage that lies in self-expression of this form is that the performer's emotions surface and he or she can then get more in touch with their own identity. As we rapidly evolve into an age of lost identity, we tend to be faddish and appear to be more and more alike. As the mass media gradually infiltrates our individuality, the result appears to be a majority of people that think in a similar fashion, have similar viewpoints and express themselves in a similar way. Conversations are becoming very predictable and repetitive. Isn't it common to hear people talking about a popular new television show or the hottest and latest movie to hit the theatres? People are tending to lose their own identity to a "Mass Identity." I am inclined to believe this has lent itself to many of the growing social problems linked to increased depression, especially amongst teenagers. Teenagers readily tackle an identity crisis as a result of their age, so is it any wonder there are so many teen suicides?

Let me assure you of something, it takes a real sense of oneself to be able to go out amongst an infinite number of conformists and Prancercise®! I was an outcast, at times; many people were just awestruck watching me. Some people would stop whatever they were doing and just gape in amazement. Other people would giggle and point, while some (especially the jealous appearing women) would act indignant and pretend to ignore me with upturned heads. Various people would cheer me on while still others who gaily imitated me would just get swept up into my positive energy. I would come upon people that appeared to be talking about and analyzing me. Several people approached me to see if I'd gone mad. An occasional groupie would inquire to see what good drugs I was on. I would observe quite a number of men encouraging their wives to try my new exercise. It's likely they were impressed with my 21 inch waist and shapely figure. Some men would just shout out "adorable," and still others would inquire if I was a Dancer or even an Aerobics Instructor. One thing was certain, nearly every one's head turned as I passed by. Yes, one would need to feel very secure with oneself to initiate such a program. Fortunately, the more I reveled in it the more secure I felt.

I must confess that my very basic non conformist nature was as much an impetus for the pursuit of my program as the feeling of self-assurance that I derived from it. I felt akin to Isadora Duncan who danced from her soul. I wasn't entrenched in any set routine or learned manner. It was for this very reason too that if someone out on the " Broadwalk" would try to imitate me, another would call out "forget it, no one can copy her." As a result of my life long rebellious, non conformist, mischievous ways, I would go out of my way to flaunt the fact that I could be so outrageous without being illegal! Whenever the police were driving by I would pretend they were pondering what they could arrest me for. It felt sensational being able to constantly disturb the public without being arrested. Ms. Duncan in her time, like myself in mine, gave many controversial performances. Some were done so in scantily covered costumes, which challenged tradition, others had political overtones. Nonetheless, disturb the public she did! Isadora, like myself, had a tremendous influence on her audience. It was mentioned that she made old men weep in their beards. I suppose that when anyone's soul is shining in what they're doing it's obvious to the public, and this cannot be manufactured. Everyone from toddlers to grandfathers were caught up in my energy, which was like a universal language, speaking to all. There are a multitude of reasons Prancercise® is the royalty of all other exercises. As I mentioned previously it attracts all genders and age groups. I actually experienced little babies turn their heads, stare, and reach out their little hands to me as I went by. On the other hand, very elderly men that were caught up in my rhythm would dance with and around me as I went by. One day one of these older fellows grabbed me and we danced hand in hand singing " Finiculee Finicula."Furthermore Prancercise® is a very practical and inexpensive mode of exercise. It requires no more equipment than a good walking or running program.

Since Prancercise® is preferably done outdoors, if you're able to do it where the air quality is good (especially by a beach or in the mountains), you will derive greater benefits than just that of normal exercise. Your body chemistry is more apt to change in this type of environment, giving you a more distinct sense of well being. It is known that the negative ions prevalent in the air of these regions, have harmonizing effects on the body. This can aid the body in obtaining a greater chemical balance internally, which can even affect one's thoughts.

Prancercise® feeds the soul, just as good food nourishes the body. Improved circulation and mental health leads to improved digestion and physical health; all are connected, and I've found that all are improved through this exercise.

Prancercise® is an individual's sport and therefore you need not rely on other players to perform it. You can exercise anytime, anywhere, and any day you choose. I have a distinct advantage living in Florida since I can exercise outdoors almost any given day. I also benefit by needing only a limited wardrobe. Loose fitting cotton clothing suits me just fine. Those living in much colder climates, may want to try layers of Danskin-like clothes that will protect them from the cold without being bulky. In extremely cold conditions, a large gymnasium or indoor basketball court is fine for prancercising. Health spas with indoor tracks are also favorable settings. In my chapter on physical gear I will discuss in more detail what you might consider wearing or using for your Prancercise® sessions.

It is my opinion, only in the understanding of the magnificent movement of the horse, can we begin to appreciate the depth of beauty and excellent means of fitness that's inherent in Prancercise®. In their wild state horses are known to have four natural gaits. These are the walk, trot, pace and run (gallop). The walk is a slow, natural, flat footed, four beat gait. It involves the horse taking each foot off the ground and then striking it at different intervals. A perfect walk executed by a horse is springy, regular and true. The trot is a two beat diagonal gait by which the front foot and opposite hind foot take off at the same time and strike the ground at the same time. The pace is a fast two beat gait by which the front and hind feet on the same side start and stop simultaneously. The feet rise very slightly above the ground and the horse floats through the air. It's a little faster movement than the trot, yet slower than the run... The final natural mode of movement for the horse is the run or gallop. This is a fast four beat gait where the feet of the horse strike the ground separately. First one hind foot strikes the ground, then the other hind foot, then the front foot on the same side as the first hind foot, then the other front foot which decides the lead. It is only through the domestication of the horse that other acquired gaits have come about. These relate to the type of horse, its breeding, and the specific schooling it's given.

Some of these other gaits are the canter, the stepping pace, the fox trot, the rack, and the traverse or side step. The canter is a slow, restrained, three beat gait by which the two diagonal legs are paired, so they produce a single beat between the successive beats of the other unpaired legs. The stepping pace is a pace usually restricted to show horses. This movement is unlike the true pace since the two feet on each side don't move exactly together. Instead it's a four beat gait by which each of the feet strike the ground separately. The fox trot is a slow, short, broken type of trot, by which the head usually nods. The horse brings each hind foot to the ground an instant before the diagonal fore foot. The rack or single foot is a fast, flashy, unnatural four beat gait, by which each foot hits the ground separately at equal intervals. This gait although easy on the ride, is hard on the horse. It's most widely used in horse shows. The final popular acquired gait of a domesticated horse is the traverse or side step. This is a lateral movement of the horse to the right or left, rather than forward or backward. This is an interesting movement to me, as it reminds me of the movement of the crab. I personally use a measure of this movement in Prancercise® and can easily identify with such movement as I fall under the Cancer division of the Zodiac. I will further explore this interesting connection later in the book. The morphology of the particular horse, his breeding and schooling, will all indicate and determine the type of movement the horse will exhibit, as well as what purposes the horse will be used for. A draft horse, for instance, is usually thick, massive and low of station. A race horse on the other hand, usually has an angular form, long legs and well-muscled hindquarters; with a closer-to-the-ground action than other horses.

Horses aren't said to dance, they're said to prance; what is the difference, you might ask? Well there really isn't a whole lot of difference, as I will illustrate. Dance is defined as: to move with the feet or body rhythmically. It's also defined as leaping or skipping, as from excitement or emotion; to move nimbly or quickly. It can finally be defined as bobbing up or down. Prance is defined as to spring or move by springing from the hind legs. It's also defined as moving or going in an elated manner, to swagger; to caper or dance. I consequently defined Prancercise® from these two definitions of Dance and Prance. Prancercise® is a springy, rhythmic way of moving forward, similar to a horse's gait and is ideally induced by elation. My Prancercise®walk A.K.A the " Prancewalk" is done in elongated strides whereby one leg is straight, knee is not bent, it remains stiff behind the body and is used to spring off this foot to propel the body forward. Next the hip rotates so that the opposite leg goes behind and is used in the same manner. The arms go back and forth and up and down graceful and rhythmic, alternating like the legs. My Prancercise®trot A.K.A. the "Prancetrot" is a combination of quick single consecutive steps one foot at a time by which you spring forward off the ground as arms go in a circular motion up and down and side by side rhythmically. My Prancercise®gallop A.K.A the "Prancegallop" is done by springing high off the ground from both your feet then one foot hits the ground again before the other, like leaping into the air. All the while the arms go backwards in a circular motion and up and down rhythmically for balance and to propel you forward.

Of all the horse's gaits known, probably the most similar to Prancercise® is that gait predominant in the "Tennessee Walker" horse. This horse's natural gait is a running walk. It's a slow, four beat gait of intermediate speed and has a smooth gliding effect. It is characterized by the bobbing of the head and the snapping of the teeth, in rhythm with the movement of the legs. These horses exhibit an easy, springy gait. From this description one can easily see this horse's gait as dance-like. This animal is moving in rhythm! The Hackney horses also exhibit movements similar to Prancercise® in that they move high off the ground. Once again, characteristics inherent to Prancercise® are springy and rhythmic movement; feet hitting the ground at different intervals; and a smooth gliding effect. Although most of the movement in Prancercise® is from the waist down as in swaying, there is arm and head movement to the rhythm of the music.

Besides enjoying the natural and acquired gaits of horses, horses have actually been trained to dance for the purpose of performing in shows and exhibits. More specific dance-like movements seen in show horses include cadence, piaffe and passage. Cadence is the use of lively, elevated steps. Piaffe is the use of a cadence trot on the spot. Passage is similar to a leap done above the ground, giving the appearance of floating. Isn't it interesting to consider that horses for over 2000 years have been imitating humans and we haven't tried the reverse?

Horse training and riding was first developed and documented by the great Greek statesman and general Xenophon. Much of the current horse training has been derived from it. Even prior to him, Simon of Athens wrote a book on horse training that was lost. Simon's principles were basically the same as Xenophon's, training through love and positive conditioning. Simon had made an interesting analogy towards the teaching of dance in illustrating his approach to horse training. He stated "If a dancer were forced By whips and spikes he would be no more beautiful than a horse trained under similar conditions."[1] Xenophon who continued to convey Simon's approach said "anything forced and misunderstood can never be beautiful."[2] When you consider these wise notions you might question all the children forced to learn and conquer the techniques of ballet. You might consider the desperate, overweight people, who force themselves to tolerate so many regimented and tedious Power Aerobics classes a week. You could readily compare these two groups to dispirited horses on which cruel methods of force were used for teaching purposes. Force is not uncommon to all these instances, in order to incur certain techniques of movement; some of them are not even based on the laws of nature (no wonder force seemed necessary)

In the sixteenth century, Grisone, the Neopolitan nobleman, introduced force into his training techniques of horses. Fortunately, a student of his, Pignatelli, was to advocate the individual treatment of the horse by humane methods. Isn't it interesting that this technique of paying attention to the individual, relates to the beauty that was to be achieved by the greatest artists of dance and other art forms. Furthermore the greatest riding master of all times, a Frenchman named Guérinère, was to assume the same approach as Pignatelli. The Spanish Riding School of Vienna to this day assumes Guérinère's techniques in the art of Classical Horse Training.

There are several key indicators used to measure success in the training of horses. A high degree of balance is evident in successfully trained horses. This relates to the number of paces the horse can keep in harmony. It's usually a characteristic that's inherent in the horse genetically through nature. Another key factor is the amount of self-control exhibited by the horse. This is seen as the horse's ability to be consistent in the performance of what's required. Finally, an important indication of a well-trained horse is reflected in the ability to understand what goes on in the mind of another creature. The horse's ability and readiness to submit to the rider's will, and to the music, is indicative of how excellently trained he's been.

In paralleling ourselves and our ability to Prancercise® to a horse's ability to be trained, is worth noting. We as thinking individuals don't need to concern ourselves (since there's no one riding us) with submitting to the will of another creature, however, submitting to the music that will generate our soul in directing our movement, is of foremost importance in prancercising. Throughout our lives we submit so much to others and can easily lose ourselves in doing so, Prancercise® is a means of getting back some of our lost identity. The movements inherent in it are easily formed by the natural movement of each individual, in rhythm, within the boundaries of the laws of nature. Perfecting balance (as horses can do), and even grace, can certainly be goals of any Prancercise® program. Just as a rider needs a decent knowledge of physiology, psychology, movement and balance in pertaining to the individual horse he's training; this knowledge pertaining to you, is very helpful in Prancercise®. Yes, there is much in common with the movement of horses and Prancercise®. I certainly incorporate cadence, rhythm and balance in my Prancercise® sessions. Furthermore, just as the horse learns to adjust to the weight of his rider, we too in Prancercise® can readily adjust to the use of ankle and wrist weights. In using these we are able to gain all the basic benefits discussed from the program, as well as further strengthening our muscles.

It is not uncommon that we see ourselves as animals in different instances. In the martial art of Kung Fu this is a common practice. In Irma Duncan's autobiography (adopted daughter of Isadora Duncan), she was referred to as a Faun girl in a photograph taken of her as a dancer. A faun being half human and half goat.[3] I personally have seen myself as a horse or centaur (half horse half human). When I was lighter in weight, I saw myself as a deer. Many American Indians see themselves as certain native animals in body and spirit. Isadora Duncan who entrenched herself in natural movement in order to develop her dances, was known to refer to a chorus segment from the "Bacchae" by

"Oh they like a colt as he runs by the river, a colt by his dam
when the heart in him sings,
with the keen limbs drawn
and the fleet foot a quiver,
away the Bacchanal Springs![4]"

Apparently, Isadora was not only focusing on natural movement, but more specifically on a horse's movement! Besides the movement of a horse and deer, I've been able to relate the movement of a crab to Prancercise®. It is deep within my very nature that I can find the answers as to why I developed this exercise. After all, I was born under the zodiac sign of Cancer. This sign is typified by a crab. The movement of the crab reflects one's personality as a Cancerian. A crab never goes forth directly, when heading towards what he's in pursuit of the crab will move backwards and especially side wards, before he'll move forwards. The underlying objective of the crab in this type of movement, is not to be suspected of what he's going after, and to ward off any impending danger.[5] Prancercise® is an exercise that incorporates considerable lateral and upward movement; you move very slowly forward, in contrast to running. Another interesting point to note, is the fact that in the creation and marketing of my program, I can honestly say I did not forge directly ahead in my pursuit of its acknowledgement. Yes, this program laid on the shelf for long periods of time while I battled the perils of mere subsistence.

Let me be more definitive now and explore the diverse reasons of why Prancercise® is similar to and different from other aerobic exercises. In doing this I'll also explore what results you might expect from it. Overall, some of the characteristics that you acquire through a Prancercise® program include an elevated spirit, increased self-awareness, a dancer's figure as well as the usual cardiovascular benefits inherent in aerobic programs. In addition, improved strength, flexibility, endurance, motor performance and coordination are all potential benefits of such a program. Like aerobic dance, Prancercise® isn't concerned with precise techniques and exact positions. These would be more indicative of modern dance and especially ballet. An overall goal of Prancercise® like aerobic dance, is aerobic benefits and muscle tone through vigorous movement over a sustained period of time. Even movement short of being vigorous, may be aerobically beneficial, providing it accelerates your heart beat for at least 20 consecutive minutes.

In Prancercise®, as in aerobic dance , there's the use of locomotor and non locomotor movement. The rhythmic sway, as well as prancing and gliding forward are locomotor movement. Locomotor movement allows you to go from place to place. On the other hand, the twisting, bouncing, swings, contractions and all movement stemming from the base or axis of the body, that doesn't propel you forward, is non locomotive.

In terms of physical fitness, you should develop increased cardiovascular endurance through improved circulation. There will be an increase in the amount of blood circulated and an increase in the number of red blood cells that carry oxygen to all parts of the body. This will occur as your body adjusts to the effects of exercise (work) and strives to recover from the increased demands thrust upon it. You will inevitably develop improved flexibility. This entails the ability to move the body and its parts through as wide a range of motions as possible without causing any unnecessary strain to the muscles. The movement in Prancercise®, like in dance, incorporates a maximum amount of flexion and extension (as in yoga), consequently aiding in flexibility. Through Prancercise®, you can develop muscular endurance; this being a measure of a muscle being able to repeat an identical movement over a time frame. Your legs should be very much a recipient of this benefit. In addition you can develop muscular strength through Prancercise®. This concerns itself with the muscular force exerted against movable and non movable objects. This is developed from the prancer's body moving against the weight of his/her own body. This strength is further improved with the addition of ankle and wrist weights. Dynamic motor performance will be improved with Prancercise®; this being the ability to maintain varying positions through vigorous movements. This is also a characteristic of the ability to balance, which is helpful in numerous activities of daily living. In varying forms of Prancercise®, you may find you're acquiring agility. This relates to being able to speedily change your body position and direction in an accurate manner. When I move from a forward prance to a backward or sideward one, I find this to be true. Other characteristics that are inevitably improved through this exercise are one's rhythm and coordination. One's ability to exercise regular or repetitious flowing movement patterns, in a smooth and accurate manner, is indicative of these combined talents. Some overt benefits you should experience from regular dedication to this exercise is the ability to obtain your perfect weight. Some intrinsic benefits should include improved respiratory and glandular function. On a psychological level, with a reduction in psychological tension, improved self-confidence, pride, and self-discipline often follow.[6] This can even lead to better grades in school.[7]

In creating your own Prancercise® program, you'll want to consider a number of important facts about fitness prior to setting your goals. Most of us aspiring athletes are all too readily aware of how overwhelming it is to sustain a self-satisfying level of fitness, yet how very easy it is to lose it. It is noteworthy, that in 2-3 weeks of inactivity, we lose approximately 20% of the fitness level we struggled to obtain. More alarming to note, is that in only one month's time of inactivity we should experience about a 50% loss of fitness.[8] In light of these facts, it is most important to maintain regular workouts, unless of course an injury prevents this.

It is believed that an individual should execute four workouts a week, in order to maintain a level of fitness. Furthermore it is believed that it is necessary to execute at least six workouts a week, to improve his/her fitness level.[9] An adequate goal for a fit or nearly fit person, would be to burn 2000 calories a week by aerobic exercise.[10] To better illustrate what this requires, consider walking or running 3.5 m.p.h. for one hour continuously, you would burn about 200 calories. Projecting further, in 1 and 1/2 hours at the same rate of speed, you'll burn about 300 calories. In one full week of burning 300 calories a day, you'd burn 2100 calories.[11] This could be achieved through any number of aerobic activities (biking, running, power–walking or even prancercising). Fortunately, we do numerous other activities of daily living that aid us in reaching our fitness goals. Some of us go dancing, some up and down stairs often, however, for top fitness these inadvertent activities cannot be considered as primary exercise. To achieve top fitness we need over 1 hour a day of aerobic exercise, with a minimal of 20 of those minutes sustained (continuously).[12]

I feel, the need for self-awareness and self-expression, should be considered as much a necessity, as a well-conditioned body. Since the 1960's, there has been an accelerated trend towards this in our society. In order to achieve this in Prancercise® or dance, you need to make your own unique qualities work for you in movement. This relates to your unique body structure, as well as your unique personality and spirit.

In general today, people are faddish and conforming more than not. People try to look, behave and dress like other people, other than themselves. No matter how hard we try to conform, no two people walk, talk, write or move precisely the same. This uniqueness within all of us is part of the beauty and essence of life. So in order to live in accordance with that beauty, doesn't it seem more natural to want to enhance our uniqueness, as in the way we move? Only you will know when you've found the right style of moving for yourself. Once you've adopted your very own form of prancercising, you will consequently obtain the most enjoyment. As time goes by, your unique form of Prancercise® will develop and grow in its form. Yes, as you build upon your style you'll be further developing your character as a person, and improving upon the way you feel about yourself.

Unfortunately, many of us who have a poor body image and thus mental image, would be aghast at the thought of going out in full view of the public and prancercising. Fortunately there are options for these people. Depending on where you live and what time of day you prefer to exercise, you can go out very early in the morning or very late in the evening, when the chances of being seen are drastically reduced. I personally spent many an hour exercising in parking garages, before I was ready to market this program. It's well within our means to take advantage of all the situations that offer us a satisfactory amount of privacy, in order for us to feel comfortable exercising. Get out there and "just do it!" as Nike's motto prompts us so well. It may not be surprising that before too long your body and unique style will be issues you'll want to flaunt. I personally found an additional reason to"just do it." At times I've found that although dancing and prancing are normally facilitated by an elevated spirit and at times it's more difficult to get started, once I do start, Prancercise® can lift me right out of a melancholy mood. Yes I'm convinced, that nothing short of a multitude of reasons, has set Prancercise® apart from all other forms of aerobics.

CHAPTER TWO

Prancercise® As an Art Form: How the Concepts of Various Revolutionary Artists Relate to the Concept of Prancercise®.

I have found that in having one's own philosophy towards life you derive more meaning out of exercise. Exercise need not be an inane series of repetitious moves, with the sole purpose of achieving an improved appearance. Thinking of and using exercise as a vehicle to express one' s daily outlook or emotions, and this lending itself to an overall reflection of one's being, is truly beautiful.

In our attempt to reach self-awareness and fulfillment we need to detach to a degree, from reality, ignoring the concerns around us, so that we can find the true meaning of our existence. This is the avenue I pursued, like many artists have done as well... Through detachment we can better reach our inner worlds, once in touch with them, we can channel ourselves through our talent, thus creating another world based on our inner one. This is not a readily accessible achievement, so many of us sacrifice this goal, in the pursuit of mere survival. One reason we are quite handicapped in artistic pursuit, relates to the fact, that our formal schooling is deficient in providing us with the raw materials that will aid us, in reaching our own philosophy of life, with an appreciation of the more real and basic values of it.

Walter Sorell, in his book "The Dancer's Image," very aptly depicts the conflict inherent in the quest of artistic expression when he states "not to drown in the masses, to be recognized, is the neurosis of our time."[1] There seems to be an emphasis in our society, on gathering and storing large amounts of information, with less concern for its relevance. Why else would programs like" Jeopardy" flourish so? How is most of this type of information significant and meaningful to our individual existence?

If movement is the essence of life, and dance the art of movement, dance is a respectful expression of movement, of life. Prancercise® is but a form of dance, it too can be seen in a similar light. It is but in the quest for the truth in self-expression, that leads the artist to transform something beautiful in life into an art form. Hence, he can not only satisfy his own need of self-expression, but satisfy the need in many (those who identify with him/her). It requires one's unique way of looking at life, in order to create art for others. It requires self-awareness, to color a picture of ourselves for others, and better illuminate ourselves to them.

So once again, how is an artist capable of totally surrendering to his/ her inner world through their art form? It is through self-forgetfulness (detachment). Ironically, the avenue to self-forgetfulness is through heightened self-awareness. This is because through a high degree of self-awareness we are readily able to know how to intentionally forget ourselves.

Poetry and dance both use rhythm to express what's beautiful in life. The concept of "Poetic Image" is what the artist creates through his own unique use of an artistic medium. A dance, a painting, a sculpture and a poem, are all various mediums. One characteristic that ideally is inherent in an art form is that it's humanly moving, it stirs one's emotions, if the poetic image of the Artist's work is powerful, it should succeed in this way.

Now you may be rightfully wondering to yourself about now, what does all this have to do with a fitness program? Well maybe you'd better re-evaluate your basic intentions for getting into shape. Aren't most people's intentions related to having a better self-image? Don't they hope to stir emotions in others when they're noticed? Well ironically, when you Prancercise® and really reflect yourself in a harmonious manner, you'll not only acquire a positive physique, but you'll likely receive all sorts of positive feedback from onlookers. People just naturally pick up on the positive emotions that this exercise helps to bring out in you. I often receive big smiles and thumbs up signals cheering me on. If you do receive as much as a smile from an on looker, then you've succeeded in bringing a moment of pleasure to this person's life, miraculously, through the reflection of your own being,…what could be more wonderful? After all, aren't so many of us driven to make only a small number of people happy in our lives? We find a partner in life and devote ourselves to making that person happy, an unrealistic goal in so many instances. First of all happiness isn't constant, it's momentary, besides, we can only assure happiness in ourselves, not others, since happiness must come from within. But to give any number of people, a moment's happiness, as they watch us in an instant of pure self-expression, what a realistic by product of our exercise sessions this is.

Using one's body in dance or Prancercise® is in a sense the purest form of artistic or self-expression. The reason for this is lying in the fact that it represents a form of non verbal communication, using nothing but the human body. In Sorell's explanation of dance as a purest of art forms he states: "The dance is the purest art it uses no artifice, no instrument for its communication but the dancer's body. It has therefore an immediacy no other art has… The body would remain a mere silhouette moving from now into then if it were not animated by something described by many poets as the flickering flame of its soul, the ultimate compressed into a moments ecstasy. In this state of rapture the dancer would extend his leap into the infinite if he would not have to become himself the very instant he is lost to it."[2]

Dance has been called "poetry in movement." It has the ability to convert what's real into something illusionary. It can thus, give additional meaning to the ordinary.

Art is something very special, just as dancing and prancing can be. How can we add to the quality of what we express? Sorell states: "Whenever we create a work of art, we should do it in the spirit that tells us this is the very last thing we would ever be able to do."[3]

I will continue to take a closer look at dance as an art form, in order to draw a deeper and wider meaning to Prancercise® (a variation of dance). In looking at dance like movement by primitive man, we can understand the most basic underlying meaning of dance better. It was primitive man who first attempted to capture rhythmic movement. The origin of the term " Ecstatic Expression," is rooted in dance. The nude body in ecstasy is a symbol of rebirth in many cultures throughout history. Bacchic ecstasy was reflected by ancient Greek artists. Many artists utilized the body in movement, as a basis for their work. Henri Maisse in the painting "Dance" illustrated Isadora Duncan's ecstatic movement. In the famous painting " Dance of Men and Women " by Goya, he displays satyr like movements of men, and maenad like poses of women. It is likely these were based on ancient Greek and Roman myth.

I find it most interesting that Goya, as did many famous artists, connect animal-like movement in humans, especially in dance like form. Isn't Prancercise® this very thing? Another artist that drew to the core of what I see as a relationship between horse and human movement, was Degas. Degas had a burning obsession with movement. He converted from the painting of racehorses to that of ballerinas. Sorell points out the relationship Degas saw in the two subjects: "In the movement, in the poses, and the relaxed positions of the little ballerinas he discovered a replica of his horses; there he found again the flawless function of the limbs, the synchronized motion of groups."[4] It was said that Degas saw women in a similar vein to animals even outside of his work. More specifically he saw much similarity between ballerinas and horses.[5]

As all forms of art lend themselves to one another, sculpture and dance are integrated in a variety of ways. The sculptor, like the dancer, creates the essence of an idea, captures a mood or thought, through gesture and pose. He expresses what lends itself to the illusion of rhythm in motion by capturing a single moment of a move. In dance, the dancer uses a series of movements and moments, differing from sculpture. There are sculptures that are derived from dancers and dances that are derived from sculptures. Isadora Duncan created many dance movements from what she saw on the ancient Greek Tanagra vases. These vases exhibited ancient Greeks in a series of poses.

Augustin Rodin, a comrade of Ms. Duncan's and a famous sculptor, used a dynamic sense in his work, which was very movement conscious. Rodin stated: "An artist should express the inner truth"[6] and he concluded, "only that which has character is beautiful."[7] This wisdom also lies at the basis of Prancercise®. By expressing one's inner truth and being, one reflects character, and thereby lends himself to reflect a form of beauty. As I've mentioned, the beauty of the physique is but one facet of the beauty to be derived from this exercise. Dance has been an expression of all sorts of life experiences and isolated emotions. We are familiar with some of the more popular ones such as wedding dances and funeral dances. Why not celebrate each day with dance (prance)? The great philosopher Nietzsche suggested this when he proclaimed: " Every day I count wasted in which there has been no dance."[8]He claimed of his writings: "My style is a dance." He saw those that defy gravity as in dance, as freer than others, as superior beings that possessed dancing souls. He saw people with "inner lightness" like dancers, as those who could rise above one's ordinariness.

Ever since childhood, I was driven to rise above the ordinary in every way I could. This could be seen in a poem I wrote at an early age:

The ocean's waves were washed unto the shore,
and from their foam were torn and formed,
the lustful lives of you and me
We spread our wings in flight to soar,
high above the mediocrity,
arriving at the gates of ecstasy

Nietzsche wrote about dancing: " Dancing in all forms cannot be excluded from the curriculum of all noble education: dancing with feet, with words ,and need I add that one must be able to dance with the pen? "[9]Nietzche, like the ancient Greek philosophers, saw dance as an inherent quality of the higher order of human behavior.

I suspect that one of the earliest true developments of Prancercise® was around 1600 A.D. At this time a great actor and dancer of the Elizabethan stage, William Kemp, developed and mastered what was known as the " Morris Dance."[10] By its description, the " Morris Dance" appears to have the seeds of Prancercise®. This particular dance was described by a leaping and tripping forward. It was also known that for publicity at this time, Kemp actually crossed the Alps doing this dance. Furthermore, he spent nine days dancing his way from London to Norwich, England. Kemp suggests characteristics of Pee Wee Herman, with whom I tried to approach with this program. It is said that in the theatre Kemp moved about doing a funny sort of a jig and wearing over sized slippers. He was a comedian/actor, who you could picture with comical manners and movement, truly unique to him. A jig is known to be a fast, springy dance, done in triple time; Prancercise® has vast similarities to such a dance.

Later in history, around the mid 1800's, Henrich Heine flourished as a great poet and ballet composer. He was famous for his ballet scenarios. He wrote the original " Faust" and "Giselle". Characteristic of Heine's writing, was that it was written in the spirit of Romanticism. Heine associated dance not only with the rhythmic expression of sensuality, but with the ecstatic state of emotionalism. These were characteristics of Dionysian themes, which worked on all the senses. In such themes, that which was seen as Pagan forces, was unleashed through movement. Isadora Duncan, one of the originators of modern dance, attempted to achieve a similar affect over half a century later. Heine believed in a dancer expressing their genuine personality through their spontaneous release of emotions. He believed this could help them achieve an image of free movement. In his opinion ballet was all too restrictive for such expression, with its set routines and positions. He also saw in ballet, Apollonian type of movement, which was in direct contrast to the free movement of Dionysian ecstasy.

Two great French poet philosophers that related poetry to dance quite well, were Stéphané Mallarmé and Paul Valéry. Mallarmé saw the dancer as a link between reality and a dream. He felt that in what the dance suggests lies what's significant in all dreams. He saw the dancer as half human and half a symbol of one less human. He saw in the dancer, an unreal quality enabling her to act as that link between reality and dream. Around the same time period (the first ½ of the 20th century), Valéry, a French poet philosopher, saw dance in a similar light to Mallarmé. Valéry spoke about dance as, "the release of our bodies entirely possessed with the spirit of illusion and drunk with the negation of our empty reality."[11] Valéry did a symposium called " Dance and the Soul," in which Socrates compares life with a dancer. In it Socrates claims: " She is a dancing woman, who would divinely cease to be a woman, if she could pursue her leap up to the skies. But as we cannot go as far as infinity, either dreaming or waking, so she, likewise, returns always to being herself again; stops being a flake, a bird, an idea; being in a word, all that the flute has pleased her to be, for the same earth that sent her out, calls her back and returns her, panting, to her woman's nature and to her lover."[12]

At the turn of the 18th century, an Italian dancer and choreographer, Viganò, invented choreodrama and instituted pantomime. He said of pantomime: "It expresses with rapidity the movement of the soul: it is the language of all peoples, of all ages and times. It depicts better than words extremes of joy and sorrow…It is not enough for me to please the eye, I wish to engage the heart."[13] Viganò composed more than 40 ballets that were performed up to 1821. At this time Stendhal was a devoted spectator and reviewer of ballets. He was also the author of dance and music books. He sought in the ballet "knowledge of the human heart."[14] Stendhal described Vigano's choreodrama: "We see it's emotional expression through pantomime with pictorial visualization through movement of groups and solo dancers[15]."Stendhal saw Vigano's objective from his miming dancers was " natural" gesture and movement. This was to ensure an enriched meaning in the performance. Stendhal described Vigano's objective with dance to be a movement of the body which was generated by the soul. This was an objective of Isadora Duncan as well as my own in Prancercise®. Theophile Gautier, a famous poet and painter of the mid 1800's, felt poems should appeal to the eye and ear, rather than just the mind. There existed much rhythm and fluidity in his writing, which could be described as musical. Being a painter as well as a writer, he wished to achieve radiance from words as well as colors and light. He wrote dance critiques and sought in what he reviewed, an overall objective of which he sought in all artists "the exaltation of beauty in life, the ultimate of ecstasy," as Walter Sorell puts it.[16] Gautier believed in the pursuit of beauty rather than virtue and believed it to lie only in nature and the arts. Gautier, and later Jean Cocteau, focused on youth and creativeness, as the roots of beauty. Both artists to combine the vitality of childishness with that of a worldly mind, in order to reflect what's beautiful and artistic. After Gautier's death in 1872, much of the Romantic Ballet waned too.

Jean Cocteau had a vast influence in capturing everyday realism onto the dance stage. He was a great poet, dancer and choreographer. He shared a similar view of the theatre to that of Gordon Craig (who will be referred to later in the book). He viewed a theatrical piece of work as, "ought to be written, presented, costumed, furnished by musical accompaniment, played and danced by a single individual."[17] Knowing the great demand on one individual this would be he saw a "friendly group," as a compromise.

Through extensive self-knowledge an artist is usually one who has taken time to focus away from the world around him, and concentrate more on knowing and expressing him/herself in terms of the world outside of them. An artist is therefore usually a leader admired and or followed by others. Self-knowledge is accumulated through avenues like art forms, yoga and close personal relationships. It also can come from long periods of solitude, away from others and outside stimuli. Periods like these comprised the most creative periods in my life. By looking deep within myself, I was able to find what was meaningful to me, in and about life. As a result of this experience, I was inspired and induced to create reflections of this meaning and myself. Art is the most personal, pure and universal language anyone can use; it crosses all language and age barriers. Dance as a form of art, can express a theme, convey an idea, or merely express a mood. There need not be a word uttered in order to convey thoughts through dance.

There are a number of revolutionary artists that inspired me in my own creative endeavors. They dedicated much of their creative work to all that's true in art and nature; helping to pave a path for those in pursuit of a higher consciousness (divine existence), mostly through their self-awareness in light of these ideals. These artists were great innovators of art and social change, who felt disdain towards academic forms.

They learned to achieve individual expression, in spite of the modes of conventional learning thrust upon them. The great international dancer and dance instructress Isadora Duncan, most assuredly, had the greatest impact on me, and consequently the development of my Prancercise® program. This dynamic dancer existed around the turn of the 20th century. She brought great new insights into the concept of dance and movement, and how they could be approached, in the purest and most natural sense. Her revolutionary approach to dance gave me an added incentive, to taking a revolutionary approach to exercise. Her ability to continuously adhere to her beliefs and ideals in dance and movement, while facing great hardships and resistance, thoroughly drew my admiration as it acted as in impetus in my own pursuit.

The doors were shut to me everywhere, although people acknowledged the merit in my program. The people who were in the positions that could promote my program, wouldn't assume the risk incurred by an entirely new venture. They required one of two things before getting involved, a portfolio of media coverage or the involvement of a renowned celebrity. The risk involved in exposing my aerobics too widely to the public, in order to gain the necessary media coverage, I felt posed a threat to the exclusivity of my concept ; especially before I had completed all my copyrighting. Soliciting a celebrity without an agent, production group, or large sums of money, left this avenue of marketing a bit too precarious for me. I finally concluded that my finest and safest avenue might be in, securing the literary interest necessary to break the ice with this program. A book on this program would not only offer me added protection on my concept, but could nicely draw together the magnitude of information I felt was relevant, which a video would not be likely to do.

In order to fulfill the mission of writing such a work, it was necessary to free my existence from the many demands on my time. I declined the objective of further enslaving myself to a full time job, to only ensure the basic comforts of most Americans. I worked for a short time as an Au Pair, receiving room and board for some child care services. Although the terrorizing cries of young children are not conducive to my creativity, the large amount of freedom I secured to make frequent trips to the public library, was enough to keep me treading water. As the need welled up in me to secure an independent, if but humble existence on my own, I sought the necessary avenues to realize this goal. I secured a large studio apartment with the remainder of my savings, and found myself living off my credit cards for a while. As my anxiety and debts were building, I even sank into a desperate affair with gambling, which nearly buried what little hope I had salvaged to survive. I fortunately endured, thanks to several of my friends, who occasionally cared for a bill or two, contending it was a charitable contribution to an artistic cause. I reached long periods through which I felt paralyzed towards writing by my anxiety towards survival. I prayed for a brighter tomorrow, when I could just wake up and write relentlessly until completion, with a trouble free mind. What a luxury to an artist such a notion surely is.

As Isadora Duncan viewed her dance, so too did I view my Prancercise® program, like a religion, with the same type of dedicated beliefs as any sacred institution. Isadora, unlike myself, was able to dedicate herself at a very early age to the pursuit of freeing her soul, and to dance. This may have been due largely to the fact, that she always had her family's stolid support behind her. There was Isadora, a revolutionary and a dancer as a young girl. Throughout my childhood I toyed with these roles, whenever circumstances permitted; however I was isolated from the means of really pursuing them. The weight of my family's interests for me, the influence the public schools had on me, and the lack of artistic affiliations around me, left me without the necessary fuel to express my true self, and find my unique purpose in life. Isadora, along with her siblings, had the unique option of being taught her basic education by her mother. She discontinued public school at a young age and pursued her artistic talents under the coaching and support of her family.

Isadora's approach to dance discouraged the vanity of self-observation. By eliminating the use of mirrors in her dance exercises, she encouraged her students to look within themselves, and dance from their heart. Without mirrors, they remained uninfluenced by the appearance of their movement. Their own hearts, and the response of the audience alone, were their guidelines. Prancercise® on the same note, is done outdoors, rather than in the aerobic's room of a mirrored health club, blazing with unnatural florescent lighting. The only measure of one's performance and progress, is how one feels during their workout. Their movement is prompted by their heart, their soul and music; as well as the reaction of any onlookers. Isadora made an important discovery when she disputed the source of all movement. It was her contention that the source of all movement was not at the base of the spine, as formerly believed, but from the solar plexus. She made this observation close to a century ago, and now there's scientific evidence to substantiate it. It is known that from the solar plexus, nerves signal the brain to generate each movement.

Isadora insisted on natural lighting, or that which was closest to it, for enhancing the environment of her dancers. She often utilized the gardens of her dance schools, as classrooms for her students. In describing that which appeared to be not from the soul she claimed, "they dance without animation, stiff, without expression, without inner feeling like automations."[18] This type of movement can also be evidenced in most aerobic or dance classes, where regimented movements and techniques are imitated by the participants, giving the appearance not unlike that of military servicemen or automated robots. In contrast, witnessing movement in dance or Prancercise® as an expression of one's self and soul, creatively, is a beautiful and uplifting experience.

John Galsworthy the famous writer, witnessed Isadora's "Duncan Dancers" at a performance in the early 1900's. He wrote in an article about them: "Each flight and whirling movement seemed conceived there and then out of the joy of being, dancing had surely never been a labor to them, either in rehearsal or performance. There was no tiptoeing and posturing, no hopeless muscular achievement; all was rhythm, music, light, air and above all things, happiness. Smiles and love shone from every one of their faces and from white turnings of their limbs."[19] Galsworthy was comparing the "Duncan Dancers" to ballet dancers where the latter were regimented in a strained and unnatural manner. Galsworthy continued to describe one of the dancers; "God knows how long she will keep it! But that little flying love had in her the quality that lies in deep color, in music, in the wind, and the sun, and in certain great works of art the power to set the heart free from every barrier, and flood it with delight."[20]Nothing man made will ever imitate or reflect the same beauty of what's natural in movement, etc... Galsworthy reinforces this by describing how he lost himself in the contemplation of beauty. At a lecture at Princeton University he stated; " How lost I was when I first looked on the Grand Canyon of Arizona; when I saw Isadora's child dancers... or the Egyptian desert under the moon."[21]

One of Ms. Duncan's greatest aims was to achieve the understanding of what was the sole rhythm of movement in nature. She felt that the way one moved was a reflection of one's consciousness and even one's social life. She felt to be of a higher consciousness, was to move lightly, freely, and with grace. Another aim of Ms. Duncan's was to free the spirits of her student/children, by freeing their bodies. She proclaimed: "A free spirit can only exist in a free body, and I want to set free these children's bodies."[22] Ms. Duncan was apt to take her work quite seriously and life lightly. I have come to a similar conclusion in my life. The reason for this is that life is saturated with hardships and grief, it's all around us, and so to be overwrought with it only paralyzes us from doing something worthwhile and bringing light to life's darkness.

Another great goal and dream of Isadora's was to build a foundation for the dancer of the future. She saw her as, "the highest intelligence in the freeist body."[23] She danced as a means of a universal language and a universal connection. She referred to the future dancer as universal when she stated:"the dancer of the future: whose dance belongs to no one nation but to all mankind." She goes on to speak of this dancer by saying," the dancer of the future will be one whose body and soul have grown so harmoniously together that the natural language of that soul will have become the movement of the body."[24] She envisioned this dancer as a symbol of a highly developed woman when she states; "She will help womankind to a new knowledge of the possible strength and beauty of their bodies, and the relation of their bodies to the earth, nature and the children of the future. She will dance, the body emerging again from centuries of civilized forgetfulness, emerging not in the nakedness, no longer at war with spirituality and intelligence, but joining with them in glorious harmony."[25]

When Ms. Duncan spoke of the dance school she wished to open she talked about her unique approach to teaching dance. "In this school I shall not teach children to imitate my movements but to make their own…the dances of no two people should be alike."[26]Two major concerns of Ms. Duncan in educating her students on dance were first of all, that the dance be entirely natural and individualized. This meant that not only was it complementary to the human body, but it also complemented the dancer's age, build, emotions, and character. Finally, she was concerned that the dance had a serious purpose, even beyond that of an art form, to help the dancer join with what is spiritual and thereby free her spiritually.

I can relate to many of Ms. Duncan's premises on dance when I approach Prancercise® and athletics. I can see the athlete of the future as one who is much more holistically developed. One who's not just a bulk of brawn, perfectly sculptured in frame, but one full of spirit, personality and an inner beauty. This beauty will radiate from a well sculptured body, giving it an irresistible glow and attractiveness, regardless of age and the perils of time.

Ms. Duncan, like myself, discovered an important insight that propelled me through my work. She discovered that man's greatest riches weren't inherent in a monetary value, but in the richness of his soul and imagination. Although I had the burdens of financial hardship and my family's expectations of me (where they hoped I would be at 40 years old), one day I truly connected with Isadora's insight

On 8/23/92 I took refuge at my mother's house, fleeing a hurricane that was entering the South Florida area. I was forced to leave my residence at a motel, located in a " High Risk " area. This was but one of the four places I moved to in just three months. I had moved all my worldly possessions four times, in order to try to find a suitable quarters, to complete this book in. Moving in with my mother during the hurricane, was in addition to the other moves, and was the one I least looked forward to.

A miserable dominating woman, even at the ripe old age of eighty, she could emotionally devastate me and lend me to depression in a matter of minutes. Upon arriving at her home, I was laden with frustrating thoughts, stemming from concerns over finding a secure and comfortable place to do my writing. I had to additionally deal with her hopeless and fatalistic outlook towards me. It was now the day prior to when the hurricane was to ravish us. It was a most exhilarating and inspiring day indeed! The gusts of fresh dry air mixed with sunshine on the fascinating landscape of the golf course. This set the stage for an exceptional session of emotional release, that would end in an uplifted spirit, only tempered by further insight, wisdom, and the tranquility that comes from the reinforcement of one's being.

There I was prancercising, releasing my emotions into the rhythm of my body to provocative music. All around me lay a marvelous maze of pathways, framed with lush greenery and brilliant colors. I entirely submerged myself in the beauty, order, and sensations of nature, with all her glory. By doing this, I honestly found renewed peace, direction, and purpose in my existence. I came home very excited, as if I had experienced a deep revelation. I realized the richness of my existence in contrast to the opulence and materialism around me. This community was entirely inundated with lavish homes that were embellished with extravagant landscapes. Here I was nearly penniless, yet, I was able to submerge myself into this privileged environment and totally enrich my soul, imagination, and spirit. I understood that the type of riches I possessed, were far superior to those that most of the residents around me were likely to have. Yes, I was vastly driven forward by this event, which arose out of my peculiar circumstances. I came home unusually excited desirous of sharing my insights with my mother. Consequently, I did something I had never done before, I insisted that mom be my audience as I researched and exposed a lot of the work I was doing on this program. I insisted that she accompany me, while I read out loud from books on the classical Greek philosophers. These books made up an integral part of my deceased father's library. After reviewing some of the prophesy of Marcus Aurelius, the great ancient Roman ruler and philosopher, I gained even greater certainty of my important mission, direction, and very reason for existence. Yes, I had finally found my truth and recognized it; what fulfillment I felt! The very core of happiness and meaningfulness, that most men desperately seek, was surely integrated in me now. So many great minds had substantiated this in their writings. Having found one's purpose, being compelled to fulfill it, allowing it to give one's life meaning and direction, and loving what you do, are all important ingredients in the recipe of happiness. Marcus Aurelius, like so many great thinkers, stressed the importance of each man to find and adhere to his unique purpose in life. As I read from any number of books to my mother, I further recognized the interrelationship of all their messages, with the message inherent in my fitness program. This program integrates the wisdom of great philosophers and meditation, as it offers one the means of enriching their soul and freeing their spirit. This is partially achieved through dance (prance) and artistic expression, in order to strive towards a higher level of self and expansive consciousness. This is such an outstanding consideration in light of the billions deficient of it. To achieve a consciousness, in tune with oneself, in order to be in tune with the planet, and surrounding universe, striving for the extended survival of them all…

Later that evening, after reading to my mother and reinforcing my purpose to myself, something even more compelling occurred. While reading Marcus Aurelius, I came upon a torn piece of paper that had been placed between two pages of the book. It was a piece of a page from a T.V. guide that my father must of torn out hastily in order to readily record a fleeting thought. My father had been dead for 15 years. He was my sole inspiration throughout my childhood. His relentless optimism and belief in me, nurtured a wealth of self-confidence throughout the first half of my life. He had scrawled out two notes on this scrap of paper, first he wrote: " It is more fruitful to read with someone else than alone." Ironically, I had done this peculiar deed with my mother that very evening. The final note my father had jotted down was the word "pertinacity." When I looked this word up in the dictionary, I found it to mean: "the ability to hold firm to one's purpose or beliefs." Oh surely I was receiving a fateful message from my deceased and beloved father. He was the only one that fervently encouraged me, all his living years. Yes, I would stick firm to my purpose of completing my Prancercise® program, and upholding my belief in the value of it. After all I was no patsy, no faddish follower of the times. In the same vein of Isadora

Duncan, I was a sort of revolutionary spirit, who through my unique perspective, wished to initiate change upon the common customs and practices. I was anticipating and hoping that this change could further enrich the lives of others.

Unlike Ms. Duncan, I was devoid of my family's pledged support in my artistic endeavors. Isadora's mother whole heartily abided by her children's recommendations in regards to their occupational directions. When Isadora suggested to her family that they go to Chicago, in order for her to further her dance career, they all consented, though they lacked the means to do so. As Fredrika Blair, the author of Isadora puts it (referring to Isadora's mother); "What they willed would be her will and their triumphs would be her triumphs."[27] In another light, one could see Isadora's mother as a horse, and her children as the riders. As I explained in chapter one, in order to obtain the ultimate ride between horse and rider, the horse must give his will to the rider's will. When such a commitment between beings occurs, there is a greater probability of success. So Isadora and her family ventured forth to Chicago, during the 1890's. In Chicago Isadora was presented as the "California Faun," in her first dance engagement there. This title seems interesting to me, since a faun is ½ man, ½ goat. I suspect her movement was being compared to that of an animal's, and of course Prancercise® bases its movement on that too. While performing at this engagement, she met Ivan Miroski, a forty five year old writer and painter, 26 years her senior. It seemed that the age barrier and their financial deficiencies, were not to impede the romance and engagement of this unlikely couple.

At this same time, Isadora was presented with another opportunity by the famous theatrical producer, Austin Daly. He offered her a part in his production of " Pygmalion " in N.Y.C., which was also to go on tour. She left Chicago and Ivan, for New York, and worked for Mr. Daly. She was forced to work for over a month unpaid, prior to the opening of the show. Having no money saved and working long hours, left Isadora hungry and exhausted most of the time. Following the tour of "Pygmalion," she received the part of a fairy, in the production of " A Midsummer's Night's Dream." The tour of this play returned her to Chicago, where she was reunited with Miroski. Although he had promised to follow her back to New York and marry her, she came to find out he was already married to a woman in London. Heartbroken, Isadora called off the engagement.

Isadora had now experienced the first of many disappointments in love relationships she would encounter. Ironically, I too experienced my first of many around her age. I was twenty years old when I broke off my first engagement. She, like myself, was quick to fall in love and always sadly disappointed.

She went on tour to London with the Daly Acting Co., returning to New York in 1898. It was at this time that she decided to build an independent acting career of her own. She began by giving dance recitals in the private homes of socialites. At the onset of Isadora's career, at the turn of the 20th century, ballet was the predominant dance form of this time period. Ms. Duncan's dance form was in direct opposition to ballet, just as Prancercise® is in direct opposition to most currently popular fitness programs. Ms. Duncan stated about ballet; "I am an enemy of ballet which I consider a false and preposterous art. False because it seemed to be unnatural in every way: it was full of set numbers, the holding poses, and meaningless starts and stops. No movement pose or rhythm is successive, or can be made to evolve succeeding action. Worse still, toe dancing ran counter to the structure of the human body: under tricots are dancing deformed muscles...under the muscles are deformed bones."[28]

This brings to mind how an argument for Vegetarianism can follow the same order. Providing we evolved from the ape, our dental structures and digestive tracts are in direct conflict with those of carnivores. This will be further addressed in chapter five.

Besides bucking the convention of dance form, Isadora revolutionized the presentation of dance in costume. She presented herself in free flowing toga like dresses, (similar to the wardrobes of classical Greeks), thoroughly exposing the dancer's arms, legs and bare feet. This boldness of her's, was to create something of a scandal throughout the respected circles she performed for..

Isadora's dances were pastoral and lyrical, weighing upon literary sources. She included in some of her programs, "The Rubaiyat" of Omar Khayyam, four quatrains to a waltz by Strauss and a piece of Mendelssohn's "The Spirit of Spring," and most important was " Ophelia and Narcissus " by the music of Ethelbert Nevin. Mr. Nevin was so pleased by her dance interpretation to his music that he set up a whole concert of his works for her to dance to. This was to have a great impact on the progress of her career. One of the few impeding factors to her progress was the infamous publicity she received in respect to her outlandish costumes. There were also some harsh critics of her Dance Art. However, neither of these, nor a devastating fire at the home of the Duncan's in 1899, was enough to smolder Isadora's determined soul. She utilized her marvelous ingenuity, to raise the necessary money for her and her family to take passage to England. She and her family endured a rough two week voyage upon a cattle boat.

Even in England, Isadora was to find, that her audiences weren't very receptive to her. As a result, she once again danced at the private parties of socialites. One of the more positive aspects that Ms. Duncan anticipated and realized in her move to London was the ability to disregard working in ballet, which had been so popular in New York. Fortunately, she happened into the right circles in London, and made substantial progress, prior to joining her brother in Paris. Her brother Raymond, had sent Isadora word of great opportunities there. Consequently, Isadora left for Paris around 1900. Once in Paris, Isadora was to meet up with her friend Charles Hallé who happened to be in Paris the same year she arrived. Mr. Hallé was the son of the famous pianist and conductor Karl Hallé, who had helped Isadora launch her career in London. It was timely that Charles should now be in Paris, he introduced her to many influential Parisians.

So it was that Isadora danced in the drawing rooms of many Parisians of high society. It was at this time that she befriended the famous sculptor, Rodin, and painter Eugene Carrière. Shortly after these important relationships unfolded, so too was Isadora to meet her most valued friend and confidant Mary Desti, who devoted her life to assisting Isadora.

As Isadora studied movement on her own, she became convinced that the center of motion for the body lay in the solar plexus not in the base of the spine as was believed. Lincoln Kirsten, the director of the N.Y.C. Ballet said that "few people ever thought or felt so profoundly as Duncan on the sources and uses of lyric movement. It is more remarkable that she should have been so methodically curious, young as she was, free from academic standard, lacking in practical background. Her growing confidence in her own technique and being suspect of the inadequacy of classical theories of dance, reinforced in her the need to seek her own way."[29] In her approach to dance and movement, Isadora took simple everyday movements such as walking, running, skipping and leaping and incorporated these into her dances and exercises. She didn't keep them as isolated movements, but created total fluidity in them as part of a series of movements. She developed movements that arose from emotional experiences, similar to Stanislavski's approach to acting. He was a famous revolutionary in the theatre and was to later carry a great friendship with Isadora. Isadora approached dance as I wish to approach exercise. A key goal of ours is to reach a stage of self-forgetfulness in order to be able to dance or exercise from one's unconscious. In order to achieve this special state, one needs to acquire greater physical and psychological self-awareness. This is more readily achieved by surrendering to music in order to get to one's innermost soul.

Isadora was to encounter other famous innovative dancers of her time, who influenced and directed her in her career. Ruth St. Denis and Loie Fuller were two of these people. Ms. Fuller for instance, was a great dancer of this era, whose unique use of light and scarves resulted in an ability to extend gesture in her performances. She exposed Isadora to influential audiences in Vienna and Budapest. In 1902 in Budapest, Ms. Duncan was to meet and initiate a relationship with Oscar Beregi, a brilliant young actor of the National Theatre. Isadora hired him to recite classical lyrics in the accompaniment of her performances. She experienced a bittersweet affair with Beregi. He was to propose to her and then retract his proposal. Isadora took ill from a broken heart. She first went to Germany, and then had a short stay in Greece, this now being 1903. She returned to Germany between 1903 and 1904 and became acquainted with the great composer Wagner's son in law, Henrich Thode. Thode was a writer and teacher; who inspired spiritual ecstasy in Isadora. Isadora maintained a plutonic love affair with Thode but had to finally break away since he was married and the relationship was to finally become too restricted.

It became inevitable that Isadora direct her energy away from love affairs; and so she was to focus instead on the opening of a school of dance in Germany. Isadora's dance was becoming enriched with the intensity of emotion she was living through. The depths of her ecstasies and sorrow were now reflected in her performances. Isadora suffered to an extreme when her love relationships didn't endure, this was probably a result of the extreme pleasure she would experience at the onset of her relationships, and it was almost inevitable that she would be severely damaged at the conclusion. Fredrika Blair in her book on Isadora explained it thus: "She had loved wholeheartedly without reserve. The rejection of her love was a terrible shock, and the thought of her past happiness only served to increase her present misery."[30] It was becoming more and more apparent to Isadora, that a man's love was not to be relied upon. Examples for her included her father's abandonment of her family and Miroski's attempt at bigamy with her. Then there were the later occurrences of Beregi's broken engagement and Thode's limited involvement with her. Blair explains Isadora's condition as a result of her dilemmas as such: " Weary of wasting her energies on a hopeless passion, she began to devote herself to a project that had long been in her thoughts this project was her school."[31] Isadora bought a house in the Grunewald district of Berlin, and sought girls between the ages of four and eight, to enroll in the school and reside there free of expense.

At this very time, Isadora was to meet the man who would most likely have the greatest effect on her and her life, Gordon Craig. Mr. Craig was an actor/director and like Isadora, a revolutionary. His aim was to change the direction of the theatre, just as Isadora's goal was to change the nature and direction of dance. Craig wished to add more realism to the theatre. In achieving this he focused upon the architecture of the set, the lighting, costumes, draperies, props and music. He aimed at creating much more interest in a stage setting than there ever has been.

Isadora and Gordon were referred to as "Twin Souls," Gordon wanted to do with the theatre, what Isadora wanted to do with dance, to represent it in the most natural and expressive manner. Here once again Isadora found herself in a complicated love triangle. Craig was attached to two other women besides Isadora, so she was to receive a very limited amount of his attention. Craig was not only married to May Gibson, but was heavily involved with Elena Meo. Elena was a violinist who had committed her life to Craig and their children. Isadora, who was also to become pregnant with Craig's child, found it most difficult during her pregnancy to receive less than the attention she needed from him. After the birth of Deidre, Isadora suffered from long periods of illness directly linked to Craig's negligible attention to her. Furthermore, as time passed and Craig felt Isadora wasn't being financially supportive enough of him, he turned cool towards her. He also felt her needs kept him from his work; this reached a peak around August of 1907. In passing through her difficulties with Craig, Isadora once again consoled herself in a new relationship with Constantin Stanislavski. This was not to become a love affair like that of Craig's, but more of a stable and inspiring friendship. Stanislavski, like Craig, had similar ideas to Isadora's. He was a famous director of the theatre, and unlike Craig, focused his attention on the acting not the setting, in order to develop greater realism for his audience. He concerned himself with how to make movements express thought and emotion through movement. He further concerned himself with how to keep emotion alive throughout repeated performances. Although Isadora took refuge in Stanislavski, from Craig, she continued to be supportive of Craig when representing him to Stanislavski. It was apparent that behind her mind was a need to acquire Craig's forgiveness for whatever she was deficient in giving him. She even became inundated with notions of finding a millionaire, who could support her school of dance as well as Craig's work. It came to be that while Isadora was working in Paris, France, in 1909, she drew the intrigue of Paris, Singer, the wealthy heir to the Singer sewing machine fortune. She toyed with the idea that she had found the solution to her dreams, in him. The oncoming love affair that she was to know with this man was to prove quite different than the tragic ones of her past. Yes, Singer would prove to be of great assistance to Isadora in the promotion of her career. Paris was the sort of man that loved to do things on a large scale. Furthermore, he liked to appear as a "Man of the Arts." Isadora was a means for him to fulfill these needs. The very mutual needs of these two, laid the grounds for a very powerful relationship.

It wasn't long before Paris purchased a large and prestigious hotel near the French Riviera, called Bellevue. He turned this over to Isadora for a school of dance. In 1911 Isadora honored Paris with a son named Patrick, who like her daughter Deirdre, was born out of wedlock. Unlike Paris, she fell short of seeing any need for being married. As a very liberated woman, Isadora was forever skeptical of the institution of marriage. This had proved to be especially true now, after paving a path of disappointing relationships. She would exclaim "People could not be bound together by contracts if they did not love one another."[32] She couldn't fathom how laws could relate to love relationships. She felt the laws that attempted to were unfounded and unjust. I find there's a great parallel between enduring love relationships and enduring exercise programs. Just as a relationship can only be certain to endure and be beneficial if it comes from the heart, so too must an exercise program. We must not base our programs on those ingredients significant to other people.

Isadora faced her greatest loss of all in January of 1913. Her daughter Deirdre 6½ years old and her son Patrick almost three years old, both met a tragic death in a car that plunged off a bridge into the Seine River. As a result of this tragedy Isadora fell severely ill that June. She suddenly felt the dire need to bear another child. Paris refused her calling her desire "frivolous," so she sought a partner elsewhere. She had a brief affair with a young Italian and became pregnant by him. Her impetuous need was only briefly fulfilled, however, when the baby died soon after its birth 8/1/14.

During this period of recovery from heartache and delivery, Isadora was to confront the outbreak of W.W.I in France. She moved out of her beloved home and school, Bellevue, in order to give the French army the use of it as a hospital for injured troops. She and her brother Raymond, became absorbed in a major relief project during the war. The two of them organized a means of supplying tools and food for many of the homeless families, whose crops and homes had been burned. They even managed to organize carpenters to erect tents for the displaced families.

I find it interesting that there was a deep seeded desire in my earlier years to pursue altruistic causes, similar to Isadora. I went to nursing school, originated a Vegetarian group, and worked as a social worker. I gradually developed the outlook that prevention was nobler than dealing with a crisis after it occurs.

Following her war efforts Isadora managed to find salvation in her dance work. She went on tour to America, Greece and Geneva. She even did her first tour of South America in 1916, gaining considerable popularity there. Preceding her tours, she went to New York where she was in a position to acquire financial support from Singer and the mayor of the city. Isadora however, wasn't satisfied with mere patronage. She insisted that the patronage be void of capitalistic motives. She consequently estranged their patronage. It was certainly puzzling to the average person, faced with trying to fathom why this artist would turn down a gift like Madison Square Garden for a dance school, on principle alone. Isadora suspected Paris wanted to profit from the publicity and revenue of such an act, so she scorned his intentions.

Although Isadora was by nature, antagonizing to many of her patrons, she was especially so with Singer. She saw him as an authoritative figure, accustomed to having his way, and this she resented. She did however, marvel in the security he offered to her, but gained satisfaction in finding ways to demonstrate her independence from him. Critics must have wondered why Singer tolerated her curious treatment of him and the answer may lie partially in a remark he once made to her, "you've got a good skin, and you've never bored me."[33] It was in the winter of 1918 that Isadora became acquainted with the great pianist Harold Bauer. Together, they did a recital, performing exceptionally well together. Although the duo became very close and were mutually inspiring to each other, Isadora was to be disheartened as usual. Bauer felt compelled to end their relationship abruptly, rather than threaten his marriage in any way.

It seems ironical that throughout my own life I was often drawn to married men. I think I felt less threatened by them, since I sneered at a life of full commitment, children and the like. These things were too time consuming, overbearing and in conflict with my own unique needs. The married men that were mutually attracted to me seemed to get caught up in my free spirited energy. I was light airy, cheerful, and not demanding to be around. The same year of Isadora's separation from Bauer, she traveled from New York to Paris. In Paris her secretary, Christine Dallies, introduced her to the distinguished pianist Walter Rummel. Isadora nicknamed him the "archangel", since he came into her life and uplifted her spirits during a time of deepened sadness. Isadora and Rummel worked well together, they moved to Cape Ferat on the French Riviera and proceeded to make much progress on their art work. But this was to be another short lived victory because much more heartache awaited Isadora. By now she was at the ripe age of forty three, ten years Rummel's senior. She appeared to be more like his mother than his girlfriend. As a result, it was not all too surprising that he would eventually fancy Isadora's young dance student, Anna. The final scenario resulted in all three parting their separate ways. As Fredrika Blair put it; "The final departure of Rummel and Anna reawoke Isadora's anguish. Each love affair after the death of her children had been an attempt to regain her equilibrium, to give her life meaning and to make it possible for her to work. Each failure subsequently plunged her further into despair. In every loss, she felt the ache of all previous losses as if for the first time."[34]

Isadora followed a pattern in dealing with her losses. Initially she preoccupied herself by doing as much as she could for others. By being absorbed with other people's needs she could subjugate her own. When she was ready to acknowledge her own pain she dealt with it by acting aggressively. After the loss of Anna and Rummel, she finally felt the compulsion to open a new dance school. She appealed to a number of countries to aid her in this endeavor. It was in 1921 that Russia proposed to provide her with a location and pupils for a school. She anxiously accepted this offer and departed for this mysterious country.

Upon her arrival in Russia, Ms. Duncan was assisted by two important men. One was the Commissioner for Education, Lunacharsky, and the other was her German interpreter, Ilya Ilyich Schneider. Schneider was part of the government's press dept. and a teacher of dance history and aesthetics, at the Russian School of Ballet. Isadora was to spend three disruptive months trying to secure a location for her school. She was finally given a location and revenues to sponsor only fifty students rather than what was required for the thousand she was promised. She further realized she would have to involve herself in a long dance tour, to create the means to continue the school.

This same year 1921,Isadora met the renowned young Russian poet, Sergei Esenin. They began seeing each other despite the huge age difference, of sixteen years. Esenin had recently been slighted by the marriage of his close friend Mariengof. It was implied that part of his attraction to Isadora stemmed from an attempt to create jealousy in his male friend. Apparently Esenin had bisexual tendencies, and this could partially explain the very turbulent affair he engaged in with Isadora.

This affair with Esenin was marked by violence and bouts of drunkenness. Esenin seemed to show Isadora as much violence as passion. It may well have been that through this affair, Isadora was attempting to forget her past tragedies and Esenin was trying to forget Mariengof. Regardless, their marriage was primarily a vehicle to secure Esenin's entrance abroad. This became necessary when Isadora had to go on tour to earn income for her school. It was most unfortunate that Isadora was hostilely received in America as a "Red," of questionable political interests. Furthermore she was forced to finish the tour alone, as Esenin involved himself in violent outbursts everywhere. He was arrested several times and finally institutionalized under psychiatric care. He was apparently rebelling against his life of walking in Isadora's shadows; for although he wasn't recognized outside of Russia, back home he held considerable recognition. It was after Isadora returned to Russia from her tour that the two separated. He reinforced the separation with a note to her saying he was in love with someone else.

I personally found myself involved with a similar character the first half of 1993. This insecure childlike man wanted foremost to control me. He wanted all my attention all the time, strictly for himself. He was severely jealous of any fame or attention I acquired personally. He like Esenin, was a most violent and dangerous drunk.

Isadora continued to tour outside of Russia. Upon returning to Moscow, she found 500 of her child/students moving in joy most naturally. She felt pleased with the evidence that her goals were somewhat met. In 1924 she made a positive impression on the Russian Party leaders with her dances based on the oppressed revolutionaries. It was the political moods her dances created outside of Russia that created hardships for her. She became trapped in Germany from 1925–27 for what they referred to as her "Political Connections." She was finally able to flee to France, but not before she experienced the death of Margot, one of her original six Duncan Dancers. Margot had been raised from childhood by Isadora and along with the other five original Duncan Dancers, had legally adopted Isadora's last name.

It was at this crucial time of financial devastation, that Isadora was offered a large sum of money to write her memoirs. Unfortunately she found herself unable to do so, likely due to the ravishing pain of confronting her past.

It was on 12/27/25 when Isadora received word of Esenin's death. They found him hung to death in the room of a hotel where he and Isadora had gone on their first rendezvous. It was an apparent suicide. Initially she had no more tears for the man, but by the spring she found herself ill an entire month from grief.

It was around September of 1926, that Vitya (Victor) Seroff entered Isadora's life, in Paris, France. Isadora was now a middle aged woman of 48 years old, Seroff a mere 23 years of age, a young Russian pianist.

They shared a love for music, and talked voraciously of memorable Russian experiences.

It was Isadora's tenacious adherence to her principles that allowed her to lose the little property she had left in her possession. She even refused a property settlement from Esenin's estate. Since she never legally divorced him she still had property rights to his assets. Her views towards marriage defied these rights, however, she believed when love was gone the marriage was gone too. As a result of Isadora's stringent loyalty to her principles, no matter how desperate her circumstances, she'd never consider raising money by any means which she considered questionable. Her behavior was described in this way: "She would never consent to cheapen her art, either by altering a program to make it more popular, or by accepting contracts to appear in music halls. She would present her dance unexpurgated in dignified surroundings or not at all."[35]

On July 8th, 1927 (exactly 25 years prior to my birth), Isadora prepared to perform for an audience she hadn't confronted in many years. She had prepared intensely for this, and selected serious musical pieces of rather grave overtones. It was as though she sensed what was to be reality, that this would be her very last performance. The performance proved to be tear jerking, and was accompanied by relentless applause. Somehow the mere coincidence that Isadora's last performance was to be on the month and day of my birth, can't help but leave me suspect as to the extent of my connection to her and her work.

As Ms. Duncan's indebtedness grew, she became more desperate and deluding, only further hastening the depth of this destruction. I personally exhibited the very same behavior with my gambling compulsion. The more desperate I became for a life of higher consciousness, of writing, art, and healthful living, the more I submerged into gambling and opposite ways. I suppose I saw gambling as an odd vehicle to fulfill my dreams or maybe just an escape from realizing how distant I was from them.

Isadora complied some of her memoirs, but unfortunately did not yet have the serial rights to them. She became subject to calling upon Singer for help. Even Singer was now most reluctant to dispense help on Isadora, as she continued to be thoroughly careless with her finances. At first Singer refused Isadora's request, when she had sent her friend Mary Desti to him in her behalf. However he did soften to her when she finally went to him in person. In "The Untold Story" by Mary, she attempts to explain Singer's sentiments."I suppose he felt sorry after I left, he always felt sorry for Isadora, but no one could cope with her extravagance, There were no explanations, no questions, simply love and tender greetings…Earthly love or desire had no part in this marvelous meeting just pity and tenderness on one side, and happiness that one was still loved on the other."[36]

It was the fall of 1927 and Isadora had become totally obsessed with a Bugatti car and its driver. She had glimpsed the two periodically, and now was totally intrigued by them. Consequently she made arrangements with the owner of the car, to have a ride in it based on her interest to purchase it. It was therefore arranged for Isadora to be picked up the evening of September 14th by the driver. Isadora's close confidant and friend Mary Desti, had acquired very negative feelings towards this arrangement and had strongly urged Isadora against it. Oddly enough it appeared that Mary's warnings only heightened Isadora's anxiousness. As Fredrika Blair quoted Isadora's response to Mary's disapproval; "My dear I would go for this ride tonight even if I were sure it would be my last. Even then I would go quicker."[36] Blair continued to describe Isadora's ruination this way;" The automobile leaped forward and then jerked to a stop and the watchers saw that Isadora's head had slumped against the rim of the door. Isadora's scarf had wound itself around the axle of the wheel, crushing her larynx and breaking her neck."

Ironically my greatest fear is that of suffocation. I've always been claustrophobic. It seems I've always struggled against a fear of suffocation that goes beyond the physical realm. It's as though I fear the suffocation of my identity, and even that of my self expression. I developed the annoying habit of vocalizing much too loudly, especially when I became excited about something. It was as though I felt that by yelling out my say so, I would ensure having had expressed myself and having been heard. I finally developed nodules on my vocal chords from this adverse habit. I actually struggled with severe Laryngitis for approximately 1½ years. I was diagnosed and told the nodules and Laryngitis was the result of voice strain over time.

Symbolically, Isadora like myself, desperately struggled and cried out for her unique self-expression; and I suspect the greatest fear of both of us was the inability to execute this. In my own pursuit of this cause, I lived a rather rebellious existence throughout my life. Besides denying myself marriage and children over and over again; I remained the black sheep of my family facing disinheritance and being disowned, by my surviving parent, for the way I chose to live. All this I gladly did in turn for executing my unique self-expression and identity. Isadora exhibited substantial self-expression in all aspects of her life, socially, politically and in her art. How I'll always applaud her.

There is a query that remains debatable and that is what remains of a dancer's art once she is deceased? In Isadora's case, there are substantial remnants… Isadora left a great impact on customs, costumes, a woman's moral standards, as well as education, throughout the ages since her lifetime. As mentioned in Blair's book; "The widespread acceptance of dancing as physically healthful and intellectually respectable, is directly traceable to Isadora."[39] She and Gordon Craig, highly influenced the direction of the theatre. As Blair continues; " Her celebration of the body and the life of the emotions and her preaching against hypocrisy, form part of the movement for freedom in the arts and in social relationships so characteristic of the twentieth century, a movement whose momentum is not spent today."[40]

Isadora's influence on dance directly, was mostly in her utilization of improvisational, unrehearsed, plotless dances coupled with the use of classical music. Isadora and her dancers practiced dance extensively, but not in a regimented, predictable manner. Their rehearsals were dancing warm ups utilized primarily to condition and loosen the body. Her format of dance would be accepted and carried forth by Fokine and many great choreographers of ballet. It was through Fokine that the English choreographers Anthony Tudor and Frederick Ashton carried on her influences. Tudor utilized her technique in the use of music and gesture that aimed at psychological truth. Ashton reflected her influence in the use of the tilt of the head and the softly curved arms, indicative of his ballerinas. Isadora's influence on ballet was considerable, however on modern dance it was yet more far reaching. Isadora's wide range of movements created numerous possibilities for the modern dancer. In the "Dance of the Furies" Isadora contorted her body, especially her arms and her fingers as she prowled, crouched and bowed her head in despair. She proceeded to rise from the floor with difficulty, in a tedious manner. Mary Wigman the great German Expressionist dancer, and whole generations of modern dancers to come drew from this approach. Even Martha Grahman's style of centering a dance around the use of the floor, found its root's in Isadora's technique. In Tchaikovsky's "Pathétique" Isadora spent an entire movement rising from a prone to an erect position. This musical piece has always been my favorite classical work.

Isadora's influence on the social milieu of her time relates to an attempt to color the image of Romanticism. This could be seen as a connection of the body and soul in opposition to industrialization, which reflected a trend of disconnection between people, their work, and the land. In light of moral standards she promoted woman's liberation which conflicted with the Victorian inhibitions of her era. In terms of dress, she prompted an increased freedom of a woman's dress and conduct. In terms of conduct more specifically, she professed a woman's right to bear children out of wedlock, and even danced pregnant herself. Through this act she condoned a woman's openness with her body and its unique beauty in it, during all its biological phases.

Some of Ms. Duncan's dance principles were drawn from the teachings of François Delsarte. He was the author of a book on " Gymnastics and Body Movement." He indicated the existence of a connection between movement and mental attitude. He focused on attitudes and the precipitating gestures derived from them. Ms. Duncan was able to influence dance with the use of expressive gesture, thereby also influencing the customs of this era to a great degree. She would elaborate on simple forms of movement giving them a natural artistic fluidity; as graceful poses passed from one another rapidly, the result was dance. It was further believed that Ms. Duncan explored the work of Genevieve Stebbins who wrote the " Delsarte System of Expression." This could account for her knowledge of the "Harmonic Pose" also derived from ancient Greek statues. It might also account for her utilization of "Artistic Statue Posing," involving movement from one pose to another in a fluid manner; "as unaffected as the subtle evolution of a serpent"[41] Movements such as these can also be evidenced in certain martial art forms such as Bruce Lee's Snake and Monkey Poses.

In presenting a more positive way at looking at the human body Isadora confronted great opposition from the typical 19th century mind set. She drew from Renaissance and Ancient Greek vases as well as paintings such as Botticelli's " Primavera." The sensuousness displayed in these works presented a unique form of sensuality linked with innocence, purity, chastity and grace not mere eroticism. Here we might see the body not unto itself, but rather as a temple which housed the spirit and intellect. Ms. Duncan's in depth research into ancient civilizations in order to form a basis for her dance had her referred to as "The Professor of Archeology."[42]

Isadora, unlike myself, saw excessive hip movement as unbecoming since it emphasized the "seat of the appetites." She questioned and broadened dance education with the realization that the source of the dancer's energy was the solar plexus not the base of the spine. She went on to explain, "the true dance must be the transmission of the earth's energy through the body."[43]It was her contention that this energy was through the solar plexus. It was established that even while she was as young as her mid-twenties, she would stand for hours with her hands over her solar plexus, attempting to receive the vibrations she felt rose from there. She suspected that these vibrations channeled the earth's energy. She felt that all energy was transmitted by waves, light waves, sound waves, etc...of which she visualized, for example, in the wind and the ocean.

Isadora influenced the format of dance by believing dances should transfer the dancer into a higher state of consciousness. She believed this could be achieved through overcoming fear, gravity and grief, and through expansive and upward gestures. She advocated the dancer's self-expression through her belief that the choreographer's work should reflect the dancer's private responses to the world.

Isadora's influence on dance education was only limited by the inability of her schools to survive their inadequate revenues and their instructor's inabilities to further her ideals of dance. Her most promising instructors would have been her original dance students, but they were more absorbed in dancing than teaching. Her unique approach to dance education was in line with Jean Jacques Rousseau's approach to it. This great 18th century philosopher suggested in his book " Emile," that removing the pupil from his parents and other such influences, allowed the tutor alone, to influence and teach them in a pastoral type of setting. The schools Isadora started were like " glorified orphanages." Within them she was the sole influence on her pupils (children) who removed from their parents and society, remained focused on their pursuit of natural self-expression through dance. From the dances Ms. Duncan composed on political and social themes of W.W.II and the Russian Revolution, she influenced many other famous innovators of dance such as Tamiris, Graham, Humphrey and Limon. Their works of the 1930's and 40's reflected such influence. Martha Graham used both Greek mythology and contemporary social themes to create her dances. Doris Humphrey used long movements of music flowing one into the other, as well as veils to extend gesture, both indicative of what Duncan had previously done. Ruth St. Denis and Ted Shawn were influenced by Duncan's use of Greek themes and symphonic music.

Tobi Tobias in a critique written for the New York Times stated: " Duncan's clear, simple lucidly constructed dances go back to the fundamentals of shape, weight and dynamics that contemporary dance has lost touch with in its pursuit of virtuosity"[44] There's been renewed Duncan enthusiasm in recent years just after 1978. There was an impressive celebration of her centennial, 100 years from her birth.

The most extensive remains of Duncan's influence on dance is seen in the development of free natural expression. Modern dance has been born from her principles, and ballet greatly influenced. As Agnes De Mille once stated:" "Before Duncan the dance was considered entertainment, she left it an art."[45]

As an innovator of art, Duncan's work paralleled some other famous innovators of art at the turn of the 20th century. One area of rapid change was in the theatre with the work of Constantin Stanislavsky, the other area of significant change was in painting, reflected in the work of Wassily Kandinsky.

Constantin Stanislavsky was credited with the culmination and enhancement of the Realistic Movement, in playwriting as in staging. He was also to lay the foundation for modern acting. Stanislavsky created detailed stage settings that accented all types of plays. His props were three dimensional and mood stimulating. He created props so detailed that certain aspects could only be detected by the actors themselves. He felt this was significant however, for if the actor could feel the mood better he'd be better able to portray it to the audience. In directing his actors he worked from inside them, actually having them reconstruct their state of mind to be consistent with the character they played. He emphasized meditation as a means of losing yourself temporarily in order to clear your mind for whatever you need to focus on. This important and productive state of mind is what I believe Prancercise® can help you reach. Stanislavsky worked at eliminating the " Presentational Style " of acting, which worked from the outside, as mask and costume were more emphasized than the acting itself.

Another vast innovator of art during this same period was Wassily Kandinsky. A Russian forerunner of painting who paralleled Duncan and Stanislavsky, as innovators of dance and the theatre respectively, Kandinsky developed much of his art work in Germany and Russia as did Duncan with dance. He formed the " Neve Kunstler Vereinigung," the New Artists Association, in 1908 representing the avant garde artists of this time. He along with Franz Marc of this association went further and formed " Der Blaue Reiter " or The Blue Rider, one of the most influential groups of 20th century art. They demanded only of its members, that they express their inner selves rather than just conforming to a style of art. Kandinsky stated: " I value only those artists who really are artists, that is, who consciously or unconsciously, in an entire original form, embody the expression of their inner life; who work only for this end and cannot work otherwise."[46]A non Munich artist of this time whose work was included in its exhibits was Picasso. For four years around 1910, Kandinsky attempted to achieve on canvas the departure of art from the objective world and the discovery of new subject matter which was based on the artist's "Inner Need."Kandinsky's search was for a universal means of communication apart from nature, one based on color, perception and sensation. He attempted to paint music. He tried to break down the barriers between music and painting, isolating pure artistic emotion. Sadler the author of a book on Kandinsky, expressed that Kandinsky's work through its lines and colors had a similar effect as harmony and rhythm do in music. Kandinsky opposed materialistic art as he felt it led to overproduction, hatred, partisanship, cliques and jealousy. Kandinsky's ideals were art for the sake of art alone, of noble and spiritual objectives, as well as for educational purposes not materialistic ones.

In considering Stanislavsky and Kandinsky in this book, I do so for several reasons. They like Ms. Duncan concerned themselves with realism in their art forms. They were interested in art as a means of self-expression with objectives beyond the ordinary, closer to the spiritual. Duncan and Kandinsky especially, saw art as a means of a pure form of universal communication, and a most honest expression of one's self. Helping you find out how to achieve this is a primary goal of this book.

CHAPTER THREE

The Right Mental Gear

By securing the best psychological format to approach Prancercise®, you're equipping yourself with the necessary "mental gear" to maximize your benefits from this exercise.

Prancercise®, unlike yoga, is a means of working through, not detaching from, one's emotions. The benefit is similar however, a more stabilized and harmonious existence. In Prancercise® you express your emotions in a harmless, nonverbal fashion; letting go of the negative ones that cause you to harbor negative feelings (energy) about yourself, your life and others. Whenever energy within you that is blocked is finally released, the result is increased vitality and comfort in your body. This directly affects your mind and your outlook on things. Dancing/prancing are vehicles that can aid in releasing these blockages.

In order to illustrate an ultimate level of being, one can achieve from a particular exercise episode, I will convey the experience of Diane Davis, a dancer/teacher and what she wrote about after a unique performance. She explained that in preparation for this performance she got very little food or sleep for days. Regardless of this, she stated she practiced more than usual. She explains how during this performance she reached an unusual state of being where she felt as though she were floating in the air, effortlessly. She remarked that after this performance she experienced a completely peaceful state for two days.[1] I personally had a similar experience when I had a therapeutic massage involving "polarity." The therapist explained how he felt tremendous energy blockages in the small of my back and proceeded to release them. I remained highly skeptical, until I put my hand several inches over the small of my back and felt tremendous heat rising from this area. Furthermore, I walked around for hours feeling like Diane Davis described, in a completely peaceful state, very alert and with increased ease and energy. In trying to compare it to something else the only thing that comes to mind is an exceptional orgasm.

Throughout history there is evidence of how dance was used to gain spirituality and strive towards divinity. Primitive dance was known to be the purest form of dance. It was used as a ritual towards worship for instance. Other uses included dancing as a celebration of fertility and as a medium for expressing one's purest feelings such as joy, love and fear. What primitive man discovered in dance was an ability to fully realize his being as well as better identify with a power greater than himself (his God).

In quoting a great religious leader Reverend Glenesk, we can see dance movement as a very spiritual and religious form of expression. "A creative work of dance opens up its audience to the fresh air of freedom simply through the use of space. If we be carried away, as it were, there seems to be a supernatural element involved. The dancers like angels, take to flight as athletes of god, possessed of forces beyond the ordinary mortal."[2] Creative Prancercise,like dance, if developed meaningfully enough, could be an uplifting even a religious type of experience for us.

Sorell sheds further light on the concept of dance movement as religious or spiritual when he says; " Some people may feel today, when technology is rampant and ready for an all-embracing dance of destruction, when the hands of the scientists try to lift veil after veil from the hidden secret of the creator, that man should revert in more than one way to himself as he was, to past simplicity. This feeling shows man unconsciously counteracting the arrogance of his waking self. Through movement he may again seek the shortest distance from his soul to his redeemer. These people feel that the free and coordinated rhythmic movement has spiritual reality and may help draw humanity together in a mystic union."[3]

Isadora Duncan was known for taking dance beyond mere entertainment to a spiritually uplifting experience as worship can be in of itself. Ruth

St. Denis around this same time, was a spiritual dance leader who envisioned a cathedral of the future. She saw it with sacred dances and a rhythmic choir with free flowing lyrical movements. St. Denis like Duncan, devoted her life to what she saw was pure and good, exhibiting this through the art of her dance. Sorell describes her quest as such: "Her entire life was a one woman's crusade against all darkness and ugliness, against disorder and disharmony."[4]St. Denis returned to the spiritual folk roots of dance, by creating researched ethnic and ritual dances that sprang from countries such as Egypt, Greece and India as well as the orient. Dionysian themes in the sculptures of the ancient Greek civilization suggested in the poses and apparent movement of the characters, physical abandonment and spiritual liberation…

In diverting from the more physical approach to harmonizing oneself, we can take a look at yoga and various other avenues of meditation. Yoga, which has been practiced for more than 3000 years, can be seen as a form of preventative medicine as well as a vehicle in obtaining peace of mind and in freeing the body, mind and spirit. In Hatha yoga there's an attempt to balance the right and left sides of the body. It is thought that through balancing the body, the mind can begin to find balance. Various yoga postures are instituted in order to find balance in the body. Once balance is obtained one's spiritual essence can begin to radiate. The more classical approach to yoga has one focusing their mind to obtain a divine consciousness through self-knowledge. It is through self-understanding that we can better understand the world, the universe and our relationship to them. New Age yoga differs from classical yoga in that it aims in bringing divine consciousness down to earth. Classical yoga aims more towards detachment from the physical realm. In new age yoga the aim is to re-enter the physical universe with a renewed body, mind and spirit. In such a way we are more able to aid others as well as ourselves in bettering the existence around us. In new age yoga there are four steps one can take in order to re enter the physical world renewed. First, it is necessary to withdraw from our everyday thoughts and concentrate our thoughts within ourselves. By doing this we can move into a more impersonal state where a higher will takes over. Next we expand up and out of one's consciousness which underlies all life. In the next step there's an accepting of our human limitations in order to bring cosmic truth down to earth. The final step involves spreading cosmic intelligence and pure love into the physical world.

In order to fortify ourselves against losing ourselves in our relationships with others in the physical world, we can follow the principles of detachment. By not being needy of others we can maintain a sense of self-reliance and not drain their energy. A divine love is one in which we can exist loving others without needing love in return. This type of love is a healthier form of love, something to strive for to reach optimal health usually acquired through some form of meditation. Through an elevated experience like Prancercise®, we can involve ourselves with others, sharing the meaning and beauty of our experiences without needing to take from them. Hence, we can detach in order to come back to the physical world, and with our new insights help enlighten others instead of secluding oneself as in classical yoga. We can detach to a degree when dealing with people that are suffering. We need to feel their suffering to some degree, in order to understand them, but not make their pain our own. Through our elevated spirit we can transmit joy, peace, light and healing vibrations to them.

Through some form of meditation we can truly lose our conditioned selves in order to find our real selves. We can lose our feelings of guilt, deceit, frustration, anger and hatred which are only the result of our defense mechanisms and the bad habits we've acquired along the way. By freeing ourselves of these we can live with a more positive energy, and create a more positive world for ourselves and others.

Meditation and detachment were guidelines for many great people throughout history. Constantin Stanislavsky instituted the principles of meditation in order to aid his acting students. He found meditation assisted them in cleansing their minds in order to adequately meet the challenges confronting them. He was known to have his students pick up tacks from the stage because this required concentration. If they weren't paying full attention to this deed, the result would be some very sore and bloody fingers. This exercise drew their minds away from their "selves" in order to clear them.

Meditation as well as the principle of detachment were guidelines exercised abundantly by the great Greek stoics and Roman sophists. From around 50 B.C. through 330 A.D., famous Roman sophists like Epictetus and Marcus Aurelius, as well as Greek stoics like Plato, Socrates and Aristotle; were among the greatest philosophers who adhered to these methods.

Epictetus, Marcus Aurelius's slave, during Aurelius's rule as Roman emperor (around 50 B.C. 30 A.D.), prophesied that isolation lends itself to uniqueness. He saw detachment as a necessary avenue to peace. He explained that nothing lasts forever, including feelings between people, circumstances and security. By deluding yourself that they do, you only direct yourself towards depression. He saw a form of detachment as humbleness. In order to move forward without anxiety we must not be desirous of something too deeply. He explained it thus; "If then, the things independent of our will are neither good nor evil and all things that do depend on will are in our own power and can neither be taken away from us nor given to us unless we please, what room is there for anxiety?"⁵ This principle helped me greatly in the execution of the Prancercise® program. For about three years I was nearly paralyzed from a combination of anxiety about the program and financial setbacks that kept me from readily following through with my goals. Fear of my concept being taken by another, and the difficulty of creating the necessary interest in the people of influence, totally froze my progress with it. Epictetus saw the purpose of philosophy as similar to the way I see meditation's purpose. He saw philosophy's purpose, " to bring his will into harmony with events; so that none of the things which happen, may happen against our inclination, nor those which do not happen be desired by us."⁶ Epictetus believed we show our knowledge through practice not words. A dear old friend of mine once summarized this so very well; " Wisdom is knowing what to do, virtue is doing it," she insisted.

From the son of Aristotle, Nicomachean, came the Nicomachean Ethics. In this work he assimilated much of what Aristotle prophesied. As did most of the philosophers of this period, Aristotle and his son saw happiness as a result of temperance of the soul; achieved through discipline, wisdom, detachment, or a combination of these. In the Nicomachean ethics there is an attempt to define happiness as; "An activity of soul in accordance with perfect virtue."[7]in adding to his definition he states; "The end toward which men strive in life is happiness. Happiness for each creature is found in the best possible performance of the function for which he is peculiarly adapted."[8]Making the time to find one's true purpose is important in achieving happiness. Meditation time helps us to achieve this. Time alone exercising, thinking or whatever it takes to create better self-awareness is the key.

Marcus Aurelius, the Roman emperor and pupil of Epictetus, wrote his summation of the principles he learned in his famous book " Meditations." He believed when one has a true purpose it is easy to act. He states: "This you must always bear in mind: what is the nature of the whole, and what is my nature, and how this is related to that, and what kind of part it is of what kind of whole; and there is no one that can hinder you from always doing and saying the things which are in accord with the nature of what you are apart."[9]He also refers to meditation by speaking of retreating or retiring into oneself for tranquility. He talks of calling one's principles to mind in order to cleanse the soul and free it from discontent, which can be the result of non-productive thoughts. He gave an example of nonproductive thoughts when he said; "waste not the remainder of your life in thoughts about others, except when you are concerned with some unselfish purpose."[10]

The great philosopher Socrates, gives much insight into the devising of a higher being. He concludes that the molding of an exceptional man requires him to be a great student of music, philosophy, and physical fitness. He realized to create harmony in one's self, there must be training of the soul and the body. He saw the harmonious soul as both temperate and courageous. He saw how nourishing but one side alone would lead to imbalance. There would either be too much softness and cowardliness or too much hardness and brutality. Similar to the views of a number of significant people I will refer to later were his views on what a true artist should be. He states: " Let our artists rather be those who are gifted to discern the true nature of the beautiful and graceful;

then will our youth dwell in the land of health, amid fair sights and sounds, and receive the good in everything; and beauty, the effluence of fair works, shall flow into the eye and ear, like a health giving breeze from a purer region, and insensibly draw the soul from the earliest years into likeness and sympathy with the beauty of reason."[11]

Just as we're coming to realize the extent of the value of music as a form of therapy, as a vehicle to self-awareness as well as pleasure, Socrates, all those centuries ago, realized what a valuable tool music was… In his discourse to Glaucon (Plato's brother) he says; " Glaucon, musical training is a more potent instrument than any other, because rhythm and harmony, find their way into the inward places of the soul, on which they mightily fasten, imparting grace, and making the soul of him who is rightly educated graceful, or of him who is ill educated ungraceful; and also because he who has received this true education of the inner being will most shrewdly perceive omissions or faults in art and nature, and with a true taste, while he praises and rejoices over and receives into his soul the good, and becomes noble and good, he will justly blame and hate the bad now in the days of his youth, even before he is able to know the reason why; and when reason comes he will recognize and salute the friend with whom his education has made him long familiar."[12]

Music is indeed a powerful vehicle in meditation and getting in touch with yourself. In more traditional forms of meditation and yoga, music can not only relieve the monotony, but can aid you in focusing. In Prancercise® when your body, mind and soul are absorbed in this activity it's far from monotonous.

In using music to assist one in meditation, instead of focusing on your pulse, your breathing or your heartbeat, you are in a sense focusing on your "Inner Rhythm." By choosing music that you are naturally receptive to, movement comes readily, you are harmonizing your body or nurturing the inner rhythm of your existence. Your inner rhythm is your energy, the energy you transmit to others, the way we all uniquely relate to our environments. Since positive thoughts lend themselves to positive results, the charisma that some of us generate is our positive energy, the result of our thoughts. By working on our thoughts, we work on our inner rhythm. From changing from within we change the impact of our environment on us. Our spirit needs to be nurtured in order to allow it to be healthy and positive. Modes of nurturing it include various forms of meditation like yoga that help us find inner peace through understanding our place in relationship to the entire universe, instead of our mere small worlds. Also by linking our own inner rhythm (a form of movement) to another form of movement (like dance) the linkage can help mold us in a more positive way. By inducing happiness through music that's akin to our own inner rhythm, we naturally find an outlet for our energy as through the movement of dance or Prancercise®.

There are all sorts of interactions with movement that can give us an uplifting feeling. Consider a race car driver becoming one with the dynamic energy of his car. Consider a rider of horses becoming one with the inner rhythm of his horse, and feeling the union of energy between horse and rider. This union of energies between car and driver or horse and rider, can be very uplifting to the person's spirit. In dance as in Prancercise® becoming one with music, uniting with this form of energy and then creating our own as the result of this union, can create a unique sustained production of positive energy which is very much self-expression. In order to induce positive thoughts and energy we'll need to utilize a specific type of music, that not only appeals to our own inner rhythm, but to our specific mood at the moment of execution. Have you ever listened to a melancholy tune but even in indulging in it we work through a bittersweet memory and derive a pleasurable feeling from this experience? By finding forms of music (mediums) that help us surface and work through emotions, we can gain a measure of peace in ourselves and subsequently happiness. When we in turn radiate peace and happiness, our environment responds back in a positive way.

In any form of meditation; yoga, Prancercise®, or otherwise, a mantra (the point of focus) can be any number of things as long as it helps you focus your mind away from the everyday concerns (static), and helps you accomplish your goals. Peace, harmony and happiness may be our ultimate goals. A more immediate goal may be clearer thinking, in order to be able to make better daily decisions.

The author of the book Inner Rhythm, discusses how 20 minutes of inner rhythm connection can be more effective than several hours of ordinary rest. A minimum of 20 minutes of aerobics is found to be necessary for the most effective benefits. Sustaining an elevated heart rate for a minimum of 12 to 20 minutes is required. For the most effective mental and physical benefits this should be your daily goal.[13]

Music has a universal quality that overrides language barriers and speaks to the soul of any human being. It's been used throughout history for medical and religious purposes. The ancient Greeks were known to treat everything from insomnia to indigestion with music. Religious institutions have included music as part of their rituals for its spiritually uplifting effect. As long as music can reach your emotions it has communicated with you pure and simply. Unlike language or mathematics you need no precise understanding of it. Health benefits have been shown to be a byproduct of music. It has been shown that changes in pulse, respiration, and blood pressure result from music. Its additionally been shown that music can increase metabolism, digestion, circulation, muscle activity and nutritional assimilation.[14] How many people do you know that don't enjoy some form of music? Even most physically and mentally disabled people can still interact and relate to music. For this multitude of reasons, the inclusion of music (especially that which connects with your inner rhythm), is of enormous benefit to an exercise program.

In the book Health and Human Nature by Paul Snyder, the author explains how people's personalities and ways of thinking (thought processes), lend themselves to illness. He indicates the importance of self-acceptance. This is one of the most difficult tasks of Americans today, who are caught up in looking for eternal youth and whatever commercialism has projected to them as attractive. How many people are born to look like the models on the cover of Cosmo or G.Q. magazines? With these images as goals, it's a wonder that more of us don't become seriously ill or just jump off a bridge from trying to change ourselves to meet these standardized ideals. Snyder goes on to depict that the profile of a cancer patient includes pessimism, depression, and lack of self-worth. He states; "Your own ability to adapt adequately to the circumstances of your life in both conscious and unconscious ways, is probably the most crucial single influence on your health."[15]He reinforces that it's our perceptions, emotions and attitudes that monitor our health to a great degree. If we could create a trophotropic response, the body would be able to return to its natural rhythm and restore its balance.

Snyder advocates the benefits of daily exercise as an alternative to meditation. He claims that exercising to the point where you're a little winded, will help strengthen the breathing muscles and allow good oxygenation of the blood. He goes on to explain that a regular increase in heart rate for sustained intervals will strengthen your heart muscle. From this kind of a routine you can expect several benefits. He concludes that you will sleep better, worry less, and develop a more positive self-image. He further suggests that there's reason to believe you'll develop a preference for a more nutritious diet, during such behavior. It is known that changes in metabolism and blood glucose levels affect one's appetite and one's desires for specific tastes. Exercise, especially outdoors in peaceful surroundings, can create unstructured forms of meditation. My own personal experiences substantiate this. I especially enjoy exercising along the ocean or through the woods.

The importance of psychological techniques in controlling one's health can be seen in trends with biofeedback. Snyder states: "The psychological techniques developed in the Eastern meditative traditions could produce the kind of control over physiological states that was being sought in the west by means of biofeedback equipment."[16] The two contrasting views of health are the mechanistic view of our Western culture and the mystical view of the Eastern culture.

The great statesman Mahatma Gandhi demonstrated many principles seen in the Eastern cultures as well as in the ancient cultures of Greece and Rome. He was adept at meditation. As an avid pupil of the " Gita "(holy scriptures of the Hindus), Gandhi saw in it an emphasis on detachment, a key element in meditation. The Gita stated: "Freedom from pride and pretentiousness, non-violence, forgiveness, steadfastness, self-restraint, aversion from sense objects, absence of conceit, realization of the painfulness and evil of birth, death, age and disease. Absence of attachment, refusal to be wrapped up in one's children, wife, home and family, even mindedness whether good or evil befall…"[17]

It is my belief that just as we struggle to be more physically fit, to be this in the true sense of the word, we need to become more aware of our bodies yes, but we need to become equally as aware of our minds and our manners perfecting them simultaneously.

Gandhi, like myself, questioned what seems hypocrisy in displays of wealth in religious and governmental institutions. He not only struggled for peace within himself, but for peace all around him. After all how enduring can our own sanctuary be if all around us there's nothing but chaos? He was educated as a lawyer and unfortunately saw difficulty in advancing without compromising his ideals. He saw doing so as poisoning his character and therefore refrained from such advancement. It wasn't until he had the opportunity to go to South Africa as a lawyer for some Porbanai Moslems that he could put his heart into his work. It is here that he fought the battle for Indian rights and won it. It was also here that he initiated what would become the famous political approach of " Passive Resistance." Gandhi realized the richness that could be found in one's soul and therefore posed the question; " What shall it avail a man if he gain the whole world and lose his soul?"[18] Gandhi viewed man as the most "Supreme Being" next to God. He believed that what was possible for one man to achieve was possible for all to achieve.

In his adherence to his nonviolent philosophy he was a vegetarian. In accordance with his beliefs of detachment and as a tool to initiate peace he often fasted. Gandhi's last fast aided civility between Pakistan and the Indian Union. It helped to put an end to the religious riots and violence in both areas, reducing the turmoil in Delhi. Gandhi believed; " Civil disobedience…becomes a sacred duty when the state has become lawless or which is the same thing corrupt and a citizen who barters with such a state shares it's corruption or lawlessness."[19] Gandhi's policies and actions made a tremendous impact on the world. He demonstrated how powerful one man can be without artillery and wealth behind him, but with his strong commitment to his principles alone, which were based on the selfless interest of all men.

The reason I have touched upon this man's life is to alert you to the tremendous power that is within you. By tapping into this spiritual power as through some form of meditation, you can achieve incredible results no matter what you are trying to achieve. The beauty is that the power and beauty that you'll possess will infiltrate all aspects of your life and the lives you'll touch around you.

We must ask ourselves are our goals for ourselves really petty, selfish and vain? If we could improve our morals and the lives of others in what we do, shouldn't we seek such? This is why I believe we need to seek our higher purposes in life. Many great thinkers have reached a similar conclusion to that of Erich Fromm who says; "Man's main task in life is to give birth to himself, to become what he potentially is."[20] Through meditative practices we can attempt to reach a higher level of consciousness for ourselves and through our example raise the level of global consciousness around us.

CHAPTER FOUR

The Right Physical Gear

In approaching Prancercise®, as you would any fitness program, you will need to prepare yourself for any adversity that could arise from it… This will not only allow you to continue your program in the most enjoyable and enduring manner; but will ensure your protection against any injuries that could otherwise occur.

One of your first considerations will be what athletic gear to wear that will lend itself to comfort, freedom of movement and insulation against injury. Furthermore, you'll want to consider the longevity of certain gear in light of the wear that is put on it. Athletic shoes and socks are undoubtedly the most difficult and important items to consider. It will almost surely take trial and error to determine the right ones for you. I personally went through 3 or 4 pairs of sneakers and countless pairs of socks before I found a suitable combination. Multiple blisters, toenail, and mild heel injuries were common for me during my first couple of months with the program. You may want to seek the advice of any sportswear authority in buying a good pair of athletic shoes with good shock absorption. Ones made for cross conditioning work the best. The problem being that athletic shoes aren't dance shoes, and because the market hasn't designed a shoe that's really suitable for this program, you'll just need to experiment with what's out there as I did.

Just the way each person dances differently the way each person prances (dance/walk or dance/run) will differ, and will determine the various pressure points to consider on our feet. There will be certain areas of your feet that will inevitably suffer more than others. For example, the insides of my large toes probably suffered the most my first month. Also around my knees and in my hamstrings I developed some strains. Through experience I found that the best way to deal with minor injuries is not to be defeated by them.

Don't forget your body will be getting use to an entirely new type of exercise, with entirely new demands being put on it. By continuing to strengthen and condition your body despite minor injuries, you'll finally fortify your body against them. Although you may look a little lame out there exercising with some minor strains and blisters, I found that its best to continue. When my blisters were worse than usual, I reverted to a normal walk and run program for a couple of days in order to allow quicker healing. When I strained the outside of my left knee I had to deviate some of my usual dance movements in order to redirect the pressure off the strain. I will assure you however, that as long as you're dealing with minor injuries, daily exercise on all areas of use will eventually condition your body to where you're nearly injury proof. I developed large callouses on the outside of my large toes of which I'm proud! It's doubtful that anyone whose even nearly fit will have any problems if they ease into a Prancercise® routine; I found myself doing excessive sessions on the onset of my program as I was so enthralled with it. By increasing the length and intensity of your sessions gradually you'll be able to monitor your limitations and avoid unnecessary injuries.

In getting back to my selection of athletic shoes, I personally ended up with a shoe that was designed not only for cross conditioning and low impact aerobics but that I customized to wear better on certain pressure points. I had a small rubber shield applied to the upper outside edge of the sole of my left shoe (ball of foot area).It's a basic guard that any shoe repair shop uses. This was one spot that was bearing the most stress, therefore wearing out far in advance of the rest of the shoe. With this minor alteration my shoes were holding up nicely after about 4 months of rigid use.

In addition to my shoes I choose to wear loose cotton clothing that absorbs perspiration well, is comfortable, allows my skin to breath, and allows maximum freedom of movement. Outside of clothing, I equip myself with a Walkman (nowadays an M3 player). This may require wearing a belt in order to secure it properly against your body. If you're wearing a pair of pants or shorts with a sturdy waistband this won't be necessary. Of equal importance to the overall protection and comfort of your body, is having uninterrupted music that induces your ideal movement as well as mental and spiritual comfort as well as pleasure. For this reason I choose to make my own aerobic compilations to accompany my workouts. I select music that induces rhythmic movement in me and lifts my spirits. Generally speaking this is music I would enjoy dancing to.

Finally, you may want to incorporate ankle and wrist weights as part of your workout gear to further develop and strengthen your muscles while exercising. In general when beginning this program most participants won't require these tools. The exceptions are those people of above average physical fitness, who have set higher than average goals for themselves. Once you've worked out with the weights, you'll find yourself quite at ease without them. Without weights you'll be more induced to move in an even more exaggerated fashion.

A very important consideration to make prior to the onset of your Prancercise® program is the prevention of injuries. This can be achieved through a combination of having the necessary knowledge of how injuries occur as well as by including modes of cross conditioning to your exercise sessions. Cross conditioning will aid your body in achieving the strength and flexibility in your range of motions so that your muscles will respond properly to prancercising. Cross conditioning is an important yet often disregarded consideration of people who work out. Not only do people get injuries as a result of this neglect, but they continue to work out with more than a minor injury. This can consequently lead to a permanent disability. In addition, you will prolong the injury and prolong work outs that will be much less satisfying to you, if at all.

In order to understand cross conditioning you should first consider the type of exercise you normally do. Next you must consider what adjunct exercises would complement your usual exercise. For example Prancercise® is a type of low impact aerobics that does more strengthening of your muscles than stretching of them. Therefore what I like to do prior to prancercising are exercises like swimming that stretch my muscles out so they'll be warmed up and better prepared to respond most beneficially to it. Other warm ups include simple stretching exercises like yoga positions. These help increase blood flow to your muscles before they're worked hard, necessary to prevent injuries. Even when you're starting to execute each Prancercise® session you'll preferably begin at a slower pace and work your way into a quicker one gradually. This is important for injury prevention since your muscles will have adequate time to warm up this way, and be capable of the necessary response and function as required.

Before I get into the detailed knowledge of injury prevention, we can consider how long, often, and where to Prancercise®. I personally try to maintain a minimum of four sessions a week for 50 minutes. This allows me a minimum of a three mile distance and over doubles the minimum time required for any real aerobic benefits (20 minutes). I find this amount of time not only is feasible to incorporate into my activities of daily living, but doesn't over tire me or stress my body in any way. I'm in fair condition and am not overly concerned with improving my condition or weight loss. For those goals you'll need to extend your sessions to six times a week for at least 50 minutes, until you reach your goals.

Where you choose to Prancercise® is of an individual preference. The options are numerous, unlike many other aerobic activities. Since you need not be concerned with having an instructor, videotapes, or other restrictive conditions, you can Prancercise® almost anywhere you choose outside, weather permitting. When weather's a factor, an indoor track in a health club or even a floor in a parking garage is not out of the question. Over the years I've prancercised on golf courses, all types of roads, jogging trails, on the beach, and actually any place I could walk. By varying your scenery, ground conditions and general environment, you are better able to remain enthused and interested in your sessions. I believe it's very physically and mentally beneficial to get a certain amount of fresh air and sunlight each day. You'll want to seek a relatively safe and clean area, ideally outside, in order to maximize the positive benefits you'll secure from this program.

In order to best prevent injuries it is best to have a basic understanding of your muscular system. By being somewhat conscious of which muscles you're using and how they normally move, you will be better equipped against injuries. In addition, you'll be better able to customize a program (selective movements), that will achieve the particular type of physical development you seek. Otherwise like myself, you can be happy with the physical development that occurs naturally, allowing Prancercise® to be more entertaining and less work.

Prancercise®

By including illustrations of the human muscular system (on the following two pages), I hope you'll be able to locate some of the muscles you'll be using within your own individual movement. I will give you an example of this by illustrating the muscles I use the most during my Prancercise® sessions.

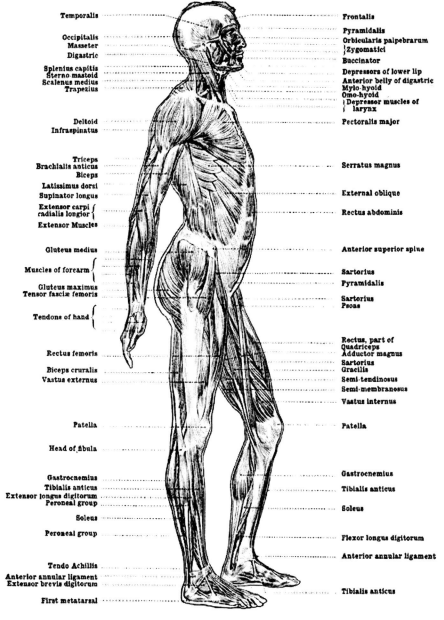

69

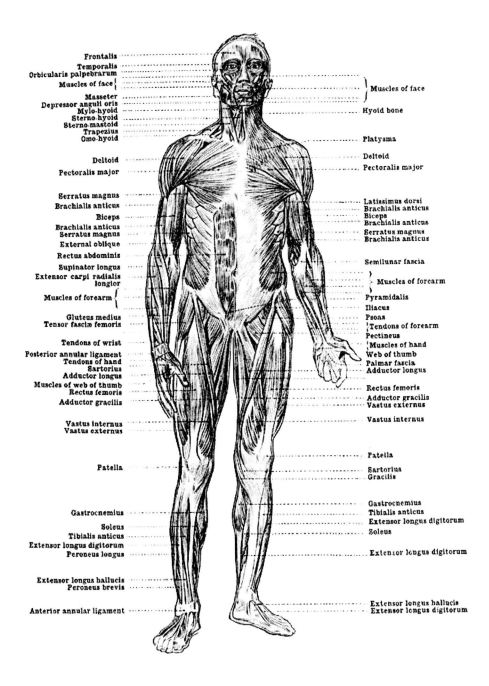

Frontalis
Temporalis
Orbicularis palpebrarum
Muscles of face
Masseter
Depressor anguli oris
Mylo-hyoid
Sterno-hyoid
Sterno-mastoid
Trapezius
Omo-hyoid

Deltoid

Pectoralis major

Serratus magnus
Brachialis anticus
Biceps
Brachialis anticus
Serratus magnus
External oblique

Rectus abdominis

Supinator longus
Extensor carpi radialis
longior

Muscles of forearm

Gluteus medius
Tensor fasciæ femoris

Tendons of wrist

Posterior annular ligament
Tendons of hand
Sartorius
Adductor longus
Muscles of web of thumb
Rectus femoris
Adductor gracilis

Vastus internus
Vastus externus

Patella

Gastrocnemius

Soleus
Tibialis anticus
Extensor longus digitorum
Peroneus longus

Extensor longus hallucis
Peroneus brevis

Anterior annular ligament

Muscles of face

Hyoid bone

Platysma

Deltoid
Pectoralis major

Latissimus dorsi
Brachialis anticus
Biceps
Brachialis anticus
Serratus magnus
Brachialis anticus

Semilunar fascia

Muscles of forearm

Pyramidalis
Iliacus
Psoas
Tendons of forearm
Pectineus
Muscles of hand
Web of thumb
Palmar fascia
Adductor longus

Rectus femoris
Adductor gracilis
Vastus externus

Vastus internus

Patella

Sartorius
Gracilis

Gastrocnemius
Tibialis anticus
Extensor longus digitorum
Soleus

Extensor longus digitorum

Extensor longus hallucis
Extensor longus digitorum

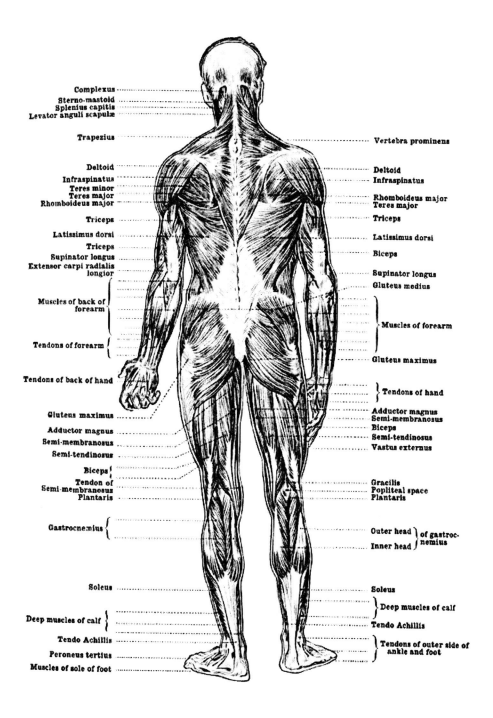

Complexus
Sterno-mastoid
Splenius capitis
Levator anguli scapulæ

Trapezius

Deltoid
Infraspinatus
Teres minor
Teres major
Rhomboideus major

Triceps

Latissimus dorsi
Triceps
Supinator longus
Extensor carpi radialis
longior

Muscles of back of
forearm

Tendons of forearm

Tendons of back of hand

Gluteus maximus

Adductor magnus
Semi-membranosus
Semi-tendinosus

Biceps
Tendon of
Semi-membranosus
Plantaris

Gastrocnemius

Soleus

Deep muscles of calf

Tendo Achillis

Peroneus tertius
Muscles of sole of foot

Vertebra prominens

Deltoid
Infraspinatus

Rhomboideus major
Teres major

Triceps

Latissimus dorsi

Biceps

Supinator longus
Gluteus medius

Muscles of forearm

Gluteus maximus

Tendons of hand

Adductor magnus
Semi-membranosus
Biceps
Semi-tendinosus
Vastus externus

Gracilis
Popliteal space
Plantaris

Outer head } of gastroc-
Inner head } nemius

Soleus
Deep muscles of calf
Tendo Achillis
Tendons of outer side of
ankle and foot

71

To begin with let me give you some general knowledge concerning muscles themselves. There are three basic types of muscles: skeletal, smooth and cardiac. The skeletal muscles are those we concern ourselves with for overall body movement. Other muscles are used by our bodies for digestion, movement of food and circulation. Skeletal muscles are utilized in our posture and the movement of our body. The use of skeletal muscles is generally of a voluntary nature by us as opposed to other muscular activity. Processes such as digestion and respiration are generally done involuntarily by certain muscle groups. Skeletal muscles are long thread like fibers that are small in diameter and therefore referred to as muscle fibers. The connective tissue that divides the muscle fibers is composed of inner and outer sheaths known as the endomysium (inner sheath), and the epimysium (outer sheath). Skeletal muscles are completely dependent on their nerve supply for function. If through injury or disease the nerves are defective, the muscles which are voluntary in movement will atrophy and not work. In the field of physical therapy there exists an attempt to stimulate muscles to work providing there is some surviving nerve units attached to the muscles. As a result varying degrees of movement can be resumed.

Since we know that muscles contract more forcibly when they're slightly stretched, it is important to stretch your muscles prior to working out (stressing them), in order to prevent injuries. Other conditions that affect the strength of muscle contractibility are adequate amounts of food, oxygen, and lower levels of lactic acid build up in the muscles. Good bodily elimination aids in keeping the lactic acid levels down. Another factor is the strength of the stimulus initiating muscle movement and the weight of the load put on the muscle. Additional factors are the temperature of the fluid that bathes the muscle as well as the muscle's size. The larger the muscle, the greater the strength of the contractions. Hypertrophy or muscle fatigue occurs when there is an excessive accumulation of lactic acid in the muscle. An example of an abnormal muscle contraction is a muscle spasm. This can be caused by one or more of the above factors which interferes with normal muscle contractions.

The names muscles are given relate to their location, the direction they take, their type of action, their size, shape, points of attachment, and the number of heads of origin of the muscle fibers. The fixed end of the skeletal muscle is its origin and the movable end being the insertion. With the exception of the face of the muscle, the origin and insertion are interchangeable (there is action and fixation at either end). The belly of the muscle is between the origin and the insertion. When a muscle cramps its often helpful to grab the belly of the muscle and apply steady pressure until the cramp is relieved.

The following muscles are some of the most predominant ones I use in my particular work outs. First of all there is the Trapezius muscle, which determines the position of the shoulders and is responsible for much of the head's movement. It's located at the front of the lower neck near the shoulder and upper back, between the shoulder and the spine. It wraps around from the back to the front of the body. The Latissimus dorsi is the muscle that moves the arm downward and backward. It's located a little less than 12 inches above the waistline in one's mid back region. It goes under the arm in the outer and upper back, and then wraps around to the front of the body. The Pectoralis major is the muscle that abducts, flexes and rotates the humerus inward. If an arm is raised it brings it back down to the side. Its located at the front of the chest in the breast area and goes to where the arm is connected to the shoulder. The Pectoralis minor works with the Pectoralis major, and is located where the Pectoralis major is. The Serratus Anterior muscles assist the Trapezius muscles in supporting weights on the shoulders and in raising the arms above the horizontal level. They're located over the outer side of the ribs in the area under your arm. The Coracobrachialis muscle assists in flexion and adduction of the arm. It's located in the front of the body in the shoulder area down over the underside of the upper arm. The Deltoid muscle is a thick powerful shield shaped muscle covering the shoulder joint and giving roundness to the upper arm, below the shoulder area. When it contracts it abducts the arm raising it laterally to a horizontal position. It aids in the flexion and extension of the arm. The Supraspinatus, Infraspinatus, and Teres minor all work in the adduction (drawing towards the main axis) of the arm. The Supraspinatus is at the crook of the Clavicle in the hollow there at the upper shoulder area in the back of the body. The Teres minor, Teres major, and Infraspinatus are at the upper, outer, side of the back and wrap around under the arm above the Lattissimus dorsi. The Teres major extends the arm and adducts it behind the back. The Biceps brahii muscle assists in the infusion of the forearm, and is a powerful supinator of the hand. That is it allows the hand to turn so the palm is facing upwards. It lies atop the Humerus bone in the arm and follows it up and down the arm from the shoulder area. The Brachialis muscle covers and protects the elbow joint and is a powerful flexor of the arm. It lies on the front side of the upper arm over the Humerus and covers the elbow joint. The Triceps brachii is a simple muscle that arises from three heads. Its located where the shoulder curves and lies on the Humerus bone. It acts as an antagonist muscle of the Biceps brachii and Brachialis. It assists in the extension of the arm and is also an important muscle in pushing. The Pronator teres pronates the hand allowing you to rotate the hand placing the palm downwards. The Sacrospinalis is the longest muscle of the body running from the sacrum to the skull. It helps in maintaining the vertebral column in an erect position. Sometimes it bends the trunk backwards to counterbalance the effect of weight at the front of the body, e.g. in pregnancy. It directly affects one's gait in the way it works and therefore is a very significant muscle in prancercising. The Iliopsoas is located from the top of the pelvis to the front of the thigh. It's a powerful flexor of the thigh and operates with it's co parts the Iliacus and the Psoas major. The Gluteus maximus forms much of the buttocks. Man's ability to walk upright is connected with this muscle. This muscle is made of many thick fibers and aids in rotating the lower extremity of the body outward, which is helpful in moving the body upward. Examples of this movement is seen in walking upstairs or in climbing… It can also be seen in springing and in leaping. The Gluteus medius and Gluteus minimus are located under the Gluteus maximus. They adduct the thigh and rotate it medially. The Sartorius is a long muscle that runs from under the pelvis diagonally over the upper front of the thigh, and down the inside of the lower thigh just above the knee. It flexes and rotates the thigh laterally and flexes the leg. The Quadriceps femoris located just above the knee, runs up the middle of the front of the thigh. It is the Rectus femoris portion of this muscle that flexes the thigh.

The Hamstring muscles are composed of three groups and lie behind the lower thigh and the knee. Their main action is to flex the leg at the thigh (the high kick), when you don't bend your knees. They also help you move your upper torso downward. The Tibialis anterior dorsally flexes and inverts the foot. It runs from the front of the foot just up from the big toe, across the front of the leg (over the Tibia) up near the knee. The Tibialis posterior runs from just below the back of the knee down through the middle of the calf. It maintains the longitudinal arch of the foot and extends and inverts the foot. The Peroneus longus runs from the lower outside portion of the calf through the bones at the front of the foot (instep area), and extends and everts the foot. The Gastocnemius and Soleus compose the muscle mass in the calf of the leg, and are inserted at the Achilles tendon (the thickest and longest tendon in the body). They're used in standing, walking and leaping. In walking they raise the heel from the ground. They allow one to stand on the tips of their toes so they're especially developed in dancers.[1] As a result of being conscious of your anatomy and physiology you'll understand the importance of warming up prior to working out.

Before I get into a more detailed account of warming up, I will reiterate the importance of other factors. Proper nutrition and rest are an integral part of the care that is needed to fortify your body against impending injury. Tired muscles can't respond properly to exercise; they'll be either too slow, quick, or jerky in their response. Sleep and rest alone will restore overcharged muscles, allowing them to relax, shorten and eliminate the accumulated wastes in them. Professional dancers can be compared to racehorses, most of them are overworked and they lack proper nutrition for the demands they put on their bodies.

The warm up session done prior to your work out should run approximately 30 minutes. This will raise your internal body temperature to between 102 and 103 degrees fahrenheit.[2] It will speed up the chemical processes in your body so that the nerve impulses can travel quicker and thus your timing and coordination are better. As you move the muscles soften and lengthen, becoming more supple and less likely to tear under stress. Walking, prancing and even gentle jogging with a springing motion that involves a change in the level of the body, with large arm movements, is especially helpful to the calf muscles before more vigorous movement commences. Warm ups will help you focus your concentration and bring your mind and body in tune with each other. They help your heart and lungs prepare for action. The warm up should be personalized; younger people may only need 15–20 minutes, older ones up to 60 minutes.[3]

There are some very helpful exercises you can do with elastic bands in order to prevent injuries in prancercising. Both static and slow stretching can be incorporated into these exercises. Static stretching is holding a muscle or muscle group in an elongated position for 30-60 seconds. Slow stretching is a gradual lengthening of a muscle group and then releasing it. Slow stretching is usually used as part of a warm up session prior to the work out session, since it loosens the muscles and prepares them for stress. Static stretching can be done periodically to help strengthen the muscles. As part of your cross conditioning program these forms of exercise will aid in one's overall fitness, endurance, performance and appearance.[4]

For the first of these exercises with elastic you need to lie on your back. Next, proceed to put a strip of elastic under the ball of your foot; now by holding the two ends of the elastic, one in each hand, stretch it from under your foot to the mid thigh area. You will be holding each end of the elastic strip on either side of your leg. Just bend the knee slightly and pull. This exercise will help strengthen the Quadriceps and the muscles of your lower leg. Proceed to do this exercise for each of your legs.

For the next exercise while lying on your back with knees bent, place a closed band of elastic over and above both ankles. Now slowly pull your legs apart while turning out at the hip joints. This will strengthen the hip abductors and lateral hip rotators.

For your third exercise lie supine (on your back) and place the elastic strip under the foot again, holding the two ends as before on either side of your leg. Now slowly point the foot pulling the band, then flex the foot and repeat. Try to do this exercise keeping the knee straight, it will help to strengthen your calf. Follow through for both of your legs.

In the next exercise you will lie on your back and place the elastic strip over the top of the middle of your foot. You'll need a partner to pull back with the strip while you pull the opposite way, flexing your foot and drawing it back towards your shin. Do this exercise for both of your legs. This exercise will help to strengthen the front of your lower leg, your ankle, and dorsi flexors.

For your fifth exercise begin from a standing position. Now place the closed elastic band around your ankles, leaving your feet slightly apart. Now slowly reach your leg backwards working the muscles along the back of the thigh and buttocks. Do this for both legs. This will help to strengthen your hip extension.

For your sixth exercise you'll once again be in a standing position. You'll place the closed elastic band around the area just above your ankles, with your feet apart, slowly move your foot upwards and sideways, with your toe slightly pointed. This should be done with each foot, it will help to strengthen your hip abductor muscles.

For your final exercise with the elastic, in a standing position place the closed elastic band just above your ankles. Now with your legs in a turned out position, with the knees pretty straight, pull one leg across and in front of the standing leg. Repeat the same with each leg. This will strengthen the muscles on the inner thigh and the hip abductor muscles.

The following exercises are done without the elastic but with the aid of other equipment. In the first one you can simply lay across your bed on your stomach, your upper torso is bent over the edge and two pillows are under your stomach. Now with your ankle weights on bend at the knees and raise your legs. This will help to strengthen your hamstrings and gastrocnemius muscles.

The last exercise I recommend for muscle strengthening and injury prevention involves the very important gastrocnemius and soleus muscles. You need to lean against a wall that has an upward slant going to it, otherwise create a slant somehow. Lean forward and slightly flex your knees in order to stretch the soleus muscle. Next, point your toes inward for the stretching and strengthening of the gastrocnemius muscle.[5]

It is important to have consistency in your work outs because muscle strength is lost at a rate of about 10% a week.

In dealing with and preventing minor injuries like weary muscles, massage can be helpful. Massage will improve circulation helping the body to eliminate wastes. Other minor discomforts like soreness or stiffness are usually due to tiny muscle spasms or tears which cause inflammation and pain. This is usually prevented through warming up. Helpful to this problem is the utilization of warm soaks and massage.

In dealing with more serious injuries there are various indications for each.[6]

Shinsplints are an injury where the muscles and tendons along the tibia become inflamed. This usually results when one's body is unaccustomed to a certain new activity it partakes in. The best treatment for this injury is rest. In addition, massage and warm water therapy have proven to be helpful. If pain ensues after ten days or so this could indicate a stress fracture and medical assistance is indicated. Muscle cramps and spasms are usually the result of overworking muscles with insufficient relaxation between exercises. These are involuntary muscle contractions that can cause considerable pain. To remedy the pain you can try grasping the painful area firmly and applying pressure to the muscle bed there. As the pain subsides, massage can break up the spasm. This can be followed by the application of heat, even a warm bath. Finally gentle slow stretching of the injured muscles will help them return to a normal condition. Foot blisters can be relieved by soaking the feet in warm Burrow's solution. Following the soak, any loose skin should be clipped away and antibiotic ointment applied. Now the blister should be covered with a sterile gauze or pad. To prevent foot blisters which arise from irritated rubbing of a shoe, perfect fitting shoes and socks should be of primary concern. Heat stress results from a loss of vital minerals from your body. You'll need to replace these minerals with drinks rich in these key vitamins and minerals like Gatorade and V8 juice. During heat stress extra rest is very important. It is common to experience chills, muscle cramping and a rapid pulse. Keeping warm and resting while your body is run down will help prevent further illness and complications.

Now we can examine modes of dealing with more serious injuries. The more common ones include strains, damage to muscle tissue, sprains and damage to ligaments. In dealing with both these injuries you'll need to stop exercising at once. Next, you'll need to apply ice to the injured area, elevate it slightly, and apply light outside pressure. A wash cloth soaked in frozen cider vinegar can be applied to the injury, this will help draw out trapped blood and fluid. The following symptoms should be signals for seeing a physician: 1) severe pain, swelling and discoloration; 2) loss of function to the area; 3) moderate pain that continues after several days. A pulled or strained muscle is usually the result of over stretching or tearing of the muscle fibers, caused by a sudden abnormal stretch or stress action. The groin, foot, ankle, calf, and lower back, can experience muscle problems usually due to an inadequate warm up. The quadriceps (muscles of the front of the thigh), on the other hand, are usually injured from over work not over stretching. In dealing with pulled or strained muscles it's important to keep the injury warm and stretch it gently each day, however, do not work out on it until it is healed. A mild strain is characterized by spasm or soreness the next day. There is no tearing of the muscle and mild careful exercise can resume. In a moderate strain where portions of the muscle are torn, you'll need to apply cold compresses and elevate the injured area for the first 24 to 48 hours, An elastic bandage should be wrapped around the injured area, and use of it should be avoided. If loss of function is ½ hour or more a doctor should be contacted. If the swelling subsides after the second or third day, soak the injured muscle in warm water or use a heating pad on it twice a day. Apply light massage just above or below the strained muscle. On or after the fifth day from the injury, begin light stretching of the muscle and wear an elastic bandage for support. A severe strain is a rupturing or pulling away of muscle from muscle, muscle from tendon, or a tendon from a bone. It's accompanied by severe pain and discoloration and a physician is indicated here. Use a cold compress and elevate it for the first 48 to72 hours. Use an elastic bandage for support. When the pain is gone you can begin stretching exercises for the injury. Sprains are a tearing of the ligaments and the surrounding tissue of a joint. They're usually the result of a sudden twisting movement. Ligaments are the tough, fibrous bands that connect our bones. Sprains must be immobilized in order to prevent further damage to them. Mild sprains are a minor twisting of the joint and usually a slight stretching of the connective tissue. They usually show only a slight loss of function and a slight amount of pain. For the first hour after the injury apply cold compresses and elevate the injury. It should also be taped or wrapped to avoid movement of it. On the second day apply heat two times a day and massage just above and below the sprained area. If it's still swollen it should remain wrapped. On the third day if the pain is gone, light exercise can be resumed. A moderate sprain results from a severe twisting of the joint. Here there's pain, swelling and discoloration, as well as temporary loss of function. For those reasons a doctor should be visited. During the first 24 to 48 hours no weight should be put on the sprain, and cold compresses and elevation should be instituted. It should be wrapped for support with tape or elastic. On the third or fourth day heat should be applied periodically. By the end of the week, you can gently move the joint. Severe sprains occur when a joint is violently twisted or dislocated. There is extreme pain, loss of function, swelling and discoloration. A physician should be seen at once so he can immobilize it into a cast. Apply cold to the injury at once, elevate it and apply a bandage for pressure and support. Put no weight on the sprain for several days, then once healed, physical therapy will help to restore the range of motion (R.O.M.).

In tendinitis, tendons (which attach muscle to bone), become inflamed from overwork or over strain. This is a common injury in dancers, especially at the knee, ankle or Achilles tendon. With this injury you should always see a doctor as soon as possible. For the first 48 hours the inflamed area should be iced. Most important is resting the injury between 1 and 3 weeks, until the pain is gone. Torn knee cartilage is usually the result of a severe strain of the knee ligaments from repeated or violent twisting. Surgery is indicated to prevent loose cartilage from catching in the knee joint. After surgery, the healing time is usually 6 to 8 weeks. Bone spurs are another common casualty resulting from frequent exercise. They are generally found in the big toe joint or in the front of the ankle. They are extra bony growths that form to protect areas of repeated stress. They are able to disappear if enough rest is given to the area. They can also be surgically removed. They are painful and restrict movement. Stress fractures are injuries that occur when chronic stress is placed on an area of the body. They're commonly found in the shins, lower back and the forefoot. They can sometimes be seen as a bump or bumps on the shinbone and can easily be mistaken for shin splints. If more than one collects on the bone it could cause the bone to break. Resting the injured area is the best remedy for them. Disc injuries include degenerated and slipped discs. Discs are the cartilage between the bones of the spinal column. They give elasticity to the back and absorb shock, thereby giving protection to the nerves near the spinal column. They join the bones of the spinal column together. A degenerated disc is one that becomes narrow and worn from abnormal stress. Helpful to this condition is a few days rest on a hard mattress, applying heat, and strengthening the supporting stomach and back muscles with exercises. If neglected, a degenerated disc can become herniated. A herniated disc is one that ruptures and the fluid from it comes out allowing the spinal nerves to be exposed to painful pressure. Surgery may reduce the pain and return as much as 75% of the original mobility, although there are no guarantees. Alternatives to surgery with these conditions include chiropractic aid and or therapeutic massage. A chiropractor may be able to release pinched nerves and restore nerve flow to an injured area. Massage can sometimes reduce muscle spasm and tension, keeping the muscles in better condition for healing.

Amongst muscle relaxation and retraining techniques are the Alexander or Sweigard Techniques. These are methods of muscle relaxation through relearning muscular habits and replacing poor ones with good ones. This can be achieved through visualization and individually supervised practice.

Meditation, acupuncture and self-hypnosis can all be used to relieve tension and promote the healing of injuries. The physical therapy approach to healing utilizes massage, hydrotherapy and similar less drastic treatments than medication and surgery. It utilizes physical remedies for defective or diseased bodily weaknesses.

Certainly the best way to deal with an injury is just to prevent it from happening. In order to prevent an injury from recurring is to analyze why it probably occurred to begin with. There are always circumstances beyond our control that could prompt an injury, but by being aware of and taking the necessary steps within our control we greatly reduce the chances of any.

CHAPTER FIVE

Eat Like a Horse and not Only Lose Weight; But Give Other Creatures a much Better Fate!

In opening a case for a vegetarian, horse type diet, I will address the prophesy of a great American Indian named Chief Seattle. Chief Seattle was an uneducated (by civilized terms) savage who possessed profound wisdom about nature. As he put it: "I will make one condition. The white man must treat the beasts of this land as his brothers. For whatever happens to the beasts soon happens to man. All things are connected."[1] Our consequences for our actions as carnivores and our mistreatment of the animals we consume is very evident. Some of our most fatal diseases can be linked to several factors, and certainly one of them being a high consumption of saturated fat (derived from meat and dairy products). We can also link bacterial diseases like Salmonella poisoning to our consumption of meat and dairy products.

How long can we deceive ourselves into believing we don't indeed suffer for our carnivorism? Aside from our own suffering, how long can we deceive ourselves into believing the animals we eat don't suffer? Many people are under the misconception that animals merely possess sensations, and that their pain has no real meaning.[2] First of all, it has been shown through research that human and nonhuman mammals have similar electroencephalograph (E.E.G.) readings. The chemistry of the Central Nervous System and Endocrine Systems are no different; and the biochemistry of the physiological and emotional states have little difference between them.[3] As far as having evidence of their intelligence, animals have continued to demonstrate their intelligence through their ability to be trained and to rescue man from danger. For us to try and justify our acts of cruelty towards creatures that cannot talk our language, yet repeatedly demonstrate their intelligence within the standardized measures we monitor them by, is surely self-deception. The argument that animals don't suffer is so full of holes that if it were true, why do we shoot horses that have broken legs or put to sleep the animals that are very ill at veterinarian hospitals? As John Robbins points out in his book "Diet for a New America", if a creature has the ability to love it surely has the ability to suffer. He further concludes that an animal that can't express its love can suffer. Providing that love is the nourishment of our souls, then just like being deprived of food causes suffering, a deficiency of love can too. In studies of animals that lack love in their nurturing, there are indications that their digestive juices remain inactive. The result of not receiving proper nutrition is retardation of all aspects of their growth. In cases of extreme deprivation, neurotic and psychotic behavior results.[4] There is an instinctive need in all creatures to give and receive love. This is surely witnessed in animals bonding with and nurturing their young. It is also evident in the act of lovemaking by adults.

Animals suffer, and they suffer for our mere pleasure; something they wouldn't do in turn to us. Animals don't suffer briefly for our consumption either, they are tortured relentlessly throughout their little lives.

Although the meat industry has made some changes over the years in offering free range and organic options, the standard processing has been as such, according to sources such as www.foodrevolution.org.

Chickens are probably consumed more than any other type of meat in our country. Their low cost and diversity of preparation, lends them to greater demand in the marketplace. Even many people who attempt to be health oriented, claim they eat chicken and fish though they've refrained from red meat. Chicken wings have become a snaking delicacy, and an increase in fire roasted chicken franchises has bombarded the consumer marketplace. Underlying the enormous desirability of this product, is the bleak reality of this poor creature's life, laden with suffering and disease.

Chickens are forced to grow up in factories, deprived of fresh air, natural light, and the type of food that's natural for them. Ninety eight percent of the eggs and poultry consumed in our country is from chickens that were raped from living the way their instincts drive them to live.[5]

No sooner has the male chick broken his way into the world, than he is sorted out because of his uselessness to the industry, and dumped into plastic bags to suffocate to death. It's been determined that the number of deaths by suffocation is ½ million a day. On the other hand the females, after but a few hours of breaking shell, are forced from their mothers and transported by conveyor belts. Their desperate cries linked to the deprivation of warmth and security their mother would give them is ignored. These females will see a very abnormal life span of about two months, if they're a broiler, instead of the normal 15-20 years for this creature.[6] Next they will be forced into cages that are stacked to the ceiling, where they are crammed together.[7] As a result of these abnormal conditions and their inability to develop their natural "pecking order," they are found fighting constantly.[8] Instead of the livestock raiser allowing a shrinkage of profits, he proceeds to cut off a part of each chicken's beak. This procedure can be compared to cutting too far into our own nails. Cutting into the soft and sensitive tissues of the bird's beak is anything but a gentle act. Further complications of this cruel act are starvation and dehydration of these poor creatures. The now abnormal beaks make eating and drinking a difficult chore.[9]

We can frame the insensitivity of these poultry producers when we hear a quote taken from one of them; " It's a damn shame when they kill each other. It means we wasted all the feed that went into the damn thing."[10] The very fact this farmer refers to the chicken as a "thing," reflects the depth of his insensitivity towards the bird. He's right in being concerned with the waste of grain, however his concern is hardly for the right reasons. The waste of our grain supply to raise livestock versus using it directly as a source of nourishment, truly eliminates the potential solution of arresting world hunger.

Layer hens, chickens used for egg production, spend the very beginning of their lives up until they can lay eggs in complete darkness. At the time they can start laying their eggs they are forced into conditions of continuous severe artificial light. This is supposed to maximize their egg production. If a layer chicken's egg production falls short of expectations the procedure of "force molting " is induced. This entails taking the hen and putting it into complete darkness without food or water for two days. This will create an artificial molting of its feathers and the growth of new ones. This procedure is used to increase the hen's egg production. If the hen survives and produces adequately, it's life is spared for two more months, otherwise it is killed for meat.

Thirty hours prior to a chicken's slaughter they are deprived of food and water as the producer feels the food wouldn't have time to turn to flesh in that time and production costs can be reduced.[11]

Another form of torture utilized by poultry raisers is the toe cutting of chicks. This is done so that their nails won't grow and get tangled in the wire of the cages they're crammed into.[12] Cramming chickens together is another way their raiser deals with the chicken's hysteria, this causes them to try to pile on top of one another smothering themselves. A standard cage is only 16"x18" for five hens.[13]

As a result of producers trying to raise the heaviest chicken possible, the bird whose bones are inadequate to support its body, finds it difficult to stand. Consequently, they huddle down developing defective feet and legs.[14] Livestock researchers are now being hired to develop a chicken genetically, without legs or feathers.[15] Producers suspect this will lead to greater profits.

From the day they're born chicks are fed antibiotics to prevent them from dying of diseases. They're treacherous and unhealthy living conditions lend itself to rampant disease in the chicken population. A chicken's diet is predominantly chemicals anyway; besides arsenic compounds and antibiotics, they're given sulfa drugs, hormones and nitrofurans, not to mention injections of dyes to add color to their flesh and egg yolks.[16] The raisers are only concerned with the weight of the chicken, its health is incidental. Chickens develop one or more of the following health problems: eye damage, blindness, sexual problems, brain damage, paralysis, internal bleeding, anemia, deformed joints and beaks, and atrophy of their bones and muscles.[17] Its little wonder that 90% of these creatures are found to be cancerous, and this is what we choose to consume.[18] A similar percent of the chickens harbor the Salmonella bacteria to which we can link much of the more immediate ill health we suffer from their consumption. Today, under pressure from consumers we see more "free range" chickens produced supposedly without all or some of these harmful conditions and additives.

There is a question that lies beyond the obvious unhealthiness of chicken consumption, it's the question of whether we assume the bad karma derived from the torture we inflict on these poor lives. After all, all things are connected.

Pigs, another form of livestock we treacherously abuse for our consumption, are actually highly intelligent and gentle animals by nature. The I.Q. of a pig actually surpasses that of a dog's. They are quite playful and good natured creatures. Their reason for rolling in the mud is to cool their bodies and deter the flies.[19]

Pigs today, like chickens, are raised in factories. They're placed in stalls so small they can barely move. The wastes from their bodies like ammonia, methane, and hydrogen sulfide, evaporates into the air around them. These vapors stay in the building emitting unbearable odors. Instead of removing this excrement, pig raisers build the pig's stall with a slanted floor, this is supposed to move the wastes into large stagnant pits. The pig whose nose is quite sensitive, is forced to breath these toxic fumes constantly. The ammonia vapors tend to poison the animal's lungs, leading to a depressed appetite and at times pneumonia.[21] Consequently the pig's diet is supplemented with antibiotics as is the chicken's. The pig's feet which aren't fit for the slanted metal or concrete floors on which they stand, develop painful open lesions in them which are prone to infection. Varying degrees of crippling in these animals is the result of the poor posture they're forced into.[22]

Sows are treated like baby machines. Normally they would produce about six babies a year, breeders have forced this to twenty a year, with goals of forty five.[23] Baby piglets are forced prematurely from their mothers only hours after their birth. The mothers stop lactating so they're pumped up with hormones to induce fertility again. A mother's sole existence is predominated with crying and mourning for her lost piglets. The piglets that would otherwise die without at least 2 weeks of sucking on their mother, are given a mechanical teat instead.[24] Here again genetic engineers are attempting to create a pig that will hold up better under the excessive weights breeders seek in them.[25] Another perverse production tactic is that of embryo transfer. Here a sow is given large amounts of hormones so she'll produce an abundance of eggs. These eggs are then removed from her surgically and implanted in other sows.[26] So many of these types of procedures are frequently the cause of the sow's death, from the excessive stress she's forced under. In contrast to the chickens that peck and eat each other from their neurotic lifestyle, pigs that become neurotic will either refuse to move, eat or drink. In more severe cases they become cannibals, biting and eating each other usually starting with the tails. In dealing with this problem, pig breeders institute the procedure of " tail docking," removing the pig's tail. This procedure causes the animal severe pain, driving them crazy.[27] In some factories looking to increase profits has gone more extreme, pigs are forced into shipping crates stacked wall to wall, floor to ceiling, with excrement from the top crates showering the pigs below.[28]

The pig's diet is more than alarming, they're fed recycled waste containing toxic residues, raw poultry, and pig manure.[29] The water they receive is from oxidation ditches that channel liquid wastes from the factory manure pits back to the animals.[30] Breeders maintain that pregnant pigs don't need to be fed for ninety days, another factor in the pig's ill health. A pig's health is similar to a chicken's, upon slaughter 80% of them have pneumonia. Other common ailments of livestock pigs include stomach ulcers, dysentery, cholera, abscesses, and trichinosis.[31] A terrible disease that killed many pigs over the years is pseudo rabies.

Some of the greatest minds throughout history preached vegetarianism. These included Plato, Tolstoy, Gandhi, George Bernard Shaw, Henry Thoreau and Leonardo Da Vinci. Ironically, these men refused to eat meat during times when meat production wasn't nearly as much of a horrifying industry.[32] It seems to me that such a wide acceptance of violence and carnivorism certainly must be linked to a high degree of ignorance on the subject.

Cattle production is another atrocity people need to look at. First of all, cattle are shipped by trucks with terrible ventilation, they nearly suffocate in the summer or freeze to death in the winter. They are also known to go up to three days without food or water while traveling.[33] Some of the cattle die from a form of pneumonia called " Shipping Fever." Breeders use a very dangerous antibiotic called Chloramphenicol to treat this fever, even though this drug can cause fatal illnesses in and of itself.[35] In the course of being shipped cattle nearly suffocate and get bruised or crippled from the bumping of the truck, especially around turns. When they arrive at a destination its common practice to dip them in a tough of insecticides... Additionally they're often castrated, de horned, branded, and injected with chemicals. In England cattle castration without painkillers is illegal, unlike in our country.[36] The castration is supposed to cause the cattle to have a higher fat content in their flesh. Following this procedure they are given synthetic hormones to replace what they would normally produce, and these synthetics have carcinogenic residues.[37] The cattle's diet is certainly no better than the chicken's or pig's. Their diet consists of sawdust with ammonia and feathers, shredded newspapers, plastic hay, processed sewage, inedible grease, poultry litter, cement dust and cardboard. This potpourri of junk is disguised by the addition of artificial color and flavors, and completed with the usual antibiotics, insecticides and hormones.[38]

The milk cows that would normally live between 20 and 25 years, now live but four years. They live their entire lives in milk factories where they are handled entirely for maximum milk production. Their sheer existence is in a concrete stall on a metal floor. The milk cow is always pregnant through artificial insemination procedures.[39] She's either chained at her neck and a portable milking machine will come to her, or she's kept in stacked cages for up to 10 months of the year and carted off 2 to 3 times a day to a milking machine.[40] The cows that are in crates can't even walk or turn around. All these cows are pumped up with hormones until their milk production stops and then they're slaughtered. The offspring of a milk cow are taken from her as soon as they're born. If the baby is a female it will become a milk cow, if it's a male it will be raised for veal. Veal raising is about a four month process.[41] The most widely practiced process is the Provimi method. This method originated in Holland and was first practiced in Wisconsin when it came to our country. The calves taken for veal are raised to get the maximum weight of tender white flesh.[42] They are put right into stalls in veal sheds. These calves who have never weaned from their mother's milk, rich in natural antibiotics, are very prone to disease. The breeder's objective in veal production is to keep the calve's muscles very underdeveloped in order to create the valuable and tender meat characteristic of veal. The calve's stall is only 22"x54" so they can barely move. They can't lie down properly, so they hunch over in a strange way with chains around their necks.[43] Their diet is purposely anemia producing so that their flesh will be nearly white in color. Their fervent need to suck is restrained by their neck chains to keep them from sucking the iron they're deprived of right out of the metal in their stalls.[44]

In place of water the calves are given a mixture of fat with surplus skim milk from the government. They drink more than they would normally of this mixture trying to quench their thirst that's not being quenched. As a result, they put the extra weight on the veal raisers are seeking in them. Another alteration to their environment is that it's always kept dark to further ensure their weight gain. Anemic and blind many of the calves contract pneumonia or enteric diseases, not surviving their four month preparation period. Consequently, breeders use two very strong and dangerous antibiotics on the calves, both linked to fatal diseases.[45] Although some people pay more for our meat when its labeled " Kosher," little do they suspect that it's not only not healthier, but it's a less humane means of slaughtering. In Kosher slaughtering the same animals are being used as in regular slaughtering however, the Koshered animal is hung upside down for 2 to 5 minutes by one rear leg before its throat is cut. For that period the animal suffers ruptured joints and broken legs in addition to the usual pain and terror. Additionally, in a Kosher slaughtering the blood vessels are removed from the animal. So that this procedure remains inexpensive only certain parts of the animal are devesseled and the remainder is sold and labeled as regular meat. About 50% of all the animals slaughtered for meat consumption are slaughtered this way, both Kosher and Non Kosher meat being derived from this group.[46]

If the future of America lies in its youth isn't it logical to be concerned with what they're taught. What may be the only education our youth gets on this subject are the twisted stories the livestock producers circulate to them. These producers take great effort to expose a very glorified picture of the lives of our livestock. They align with the National Dairy Council to distribute to schools colorful charts of the four food groups.[47] The four food groups stress the consumption of meat and dairy products. A child maintains some sort of distorted concept of Borden's contented cow " Elsie," softly reminding him to drink his milk in order to grow big and strong. Children are blatantly cultivated to become meat eaters, so that the meat and dairy industries can continue to realize their usual profits. Although children are brainwashed to believe their health is linked to meat and dairy products, it's very interesting to view the facts that question this belief system. The people belonging to the Hunza tribe from the Himalayas in North Pakistan live on a diet that's 98.5% void of meat and dairy products. These people have an amazing life expectancy of between ninety and one hundred years.[48] On the other hand the Eskimos are a people who consume the highest percentage of meat, their life expectancy is merely thirty years.[49]

Studies done by the Yale Medical School have determined that greater strength and endurance is linked to those who partake in a vegetarian diet.[50] This finding is further substantiated when we look at vegetarian athletes. Dave Scott who won the Ironman competition four times, three of them in a row, is a vegetarian.[51] What's even more amazing is that no one else at that time had won it more than once. Scott majored in exercise physiology and is thought by many to be one of the fittest men that ever existed. These facts are far from surprising to me when I look at horses, one of the strongest and most enduring animals in the world, they are true vegetarians. Another outstanding human athlete of a vegetarian orientation is Edwin Moses. Moses, an Olympic gold medalist was also the 1984 Sportsman of the Year. He was undefeated for eight years at the 400 meter hurdles. You would hardly call him and Scott "Wimpy Vegetarians." The list of outstanding vegetarian athletes is lengthy, so the argument that we must consume meat for strength and a well-balanced diet appears to be mere rhetoric. Studies have shown that 95%of all meat eaters that change to a vegetarian diet experience increased energy and well being.[52] The exceptions appear to relate to one's own individual body chemistry which could work and prevail differently than the majority of people.

The misleading suggestions that we need meat to fulfill our protein requirements are ridiculous… Our protein requirements 2.5–10% of our caloric intake, can easily be supplied by vegetables grains and beans.[53] Why 35% of the calories from soybeans alone is protein. An amazing 49% of the calories from spinach are protein. On the other hand osteoporosis is linked to excessive intake of protein.[54] Meat and dairy products are the most acid forming foods. Calcium is used by the body to buffer the blood when it's too acidic. The body will even draw calcium from the bones in order to buffer very high blood acidity (common in meat eaters), the result of this bone leaching is osteoporosis. Another complication from too much animal protein is kidney stones. The excessive calcium that ends up in the blood of meat eaters, eventually end up in the kidneys which can lead to stones

It has been shown that increased meat and saturated fat intake correlates with cancer, particularly colon cancer. While a diet high in fiber (vacant in meat and dairy products), is known to reduce the risk of cancer, especially of the colon.[55]

It is suspected that premature puberty in our youth relates to an increase in the hormonal levels of adolescents and children. This is likely to be linked to the extremely high hormonal levels found in our meat and dairy products. Breeders liberally inject these into the livestock in order to spur their growth. Women in our country are experiencing an abundance of breast and cervical cancer. Doctors won't deny this correlates with excessively high estrogen levels. Why would women be having these abnormally high levels? With the ingestion of additional hormones from meat and dairy products as well as the rampant usage of birth control pills we can begin to see the answers

Diabetes is partially linked to high fat and sugar diets. It is further known that this disease has been regulated by a more vegetarian diet to the point that 30% less insulin is required for treatment.[57] There are a multitude of other health problems related to meat and dairy consumption these are: hypoglycemia, ulcers, constipation, hemorrhoids, diverticulosis, obesity, high blood pressure, heart conditions, gall stones, and food poisoning especially from Salmonella bacteria. Alarming is how Salmonella poisoning is becoming harder to treat. The reason for this difficulty seems to be linked to the fact these bacteria are becoming increasingly resistant to many antibiotics. It's suspected this occurs when the livestock are given antibiotics by the breeders.[58] The hazards of consuming meat and dairy products don't stop here, the toxicity of a number of drugs and pesticides used on livestock is truly criminal. The hormone D.E.S. has been used periodically even though its use is illegal. D.E.S. is a confirmed carcinogen and when it's not used other dangerous hormones like Steer-oid, Ralgro, Comudose and Synover replace it.[59] Then there's the carcinogenic pesticides that don't break down for decades like D.D.T., Aldrin, Kepone, Dieldrin, Chloradane, Heptachlor, Endrin, Mirex, P.C.B.'s and Toxaphene that are used on our livestock.[60] P.C.B.'s (chlorinated hydrocarbons) found in fish and fish meal, is fed to our livestock. Fish, which compound toxins from the environment they live in, can create toxicity up to 9 million times the levels originally occurring around them.[61]

In the 1970's and 80's there was an abundance of recalled food from the Campbell and Banquet food companies, when the levels of hormones and pesticides found in their meat and dairy products were found to be at severely dangerous levels. Unfortunately payoffs by companies to government officials often times quash the limited protection consumers occupy.

Unfortunately, we don't alone suffer the consequences of what we choose to eat. Babies born to mothers who have these stored toxins in their systems, have the toxins passed on to them as in the milk they nurse them with. Even if they don't nurse their babies themselves, babies suffer from birth defects that are caused by chemicals livestock have acquired. There lies a no win argument in whether or not to breast feed an infant. The E.P.A. determined that the average American infant that's been breast fed takes in approximately 9x's the levels allowed of Dieldrin, a powerful carcinogen and about 10x's the allowance of P.C.B.'s[62] On the other hand, by not breast feeding, the infant can't receive the antibiotics it needs from its mother to protect itself from illness. In preparation for having a child we must keep this information in mind. We must also consider that on the part of the male, their sperm is damaged by toxins and this too is a factor in his offspring. Just from knowing that D.N.A. itself can be altered by toxins, it's not unreasonable to suspect that cancer, sterility and birth defects are the dangerous consequences of ingesting them.

Besides our own direct suffering and that of our offspring, we are destroying the planet itself and its other inhabitants by the mere act of choosing our diets. Yes indeed, all things are connected.

It has been determined that the livestock of the United States consumes enough grain and soybeans to feed five times the entire human population of our country![63] If we ate the grain directly, we would receive ten times the calories as otherwise.[64] We actually lose 90% of the amount of food that would otherwise be available. The grain wasted on livestock versus our direct consumption of it breaks down to a loss of 96% of the calories, 100% of the fiber and 100% of the carbohydrates.[65] Knowing that a child dies of starvation every 2 seconds, makes it difficult for me to support a meat based diet.[66]

There exists a theory that violence and war are by products of meat consumption. As a result of limited resources our fears build that we won't have enough of them. With compounding fear there tends to be more concern about territorial rights. War is an outgrowth of these concerns, it can be assumed that by reducing these concerns we could reduce the likelihood of war and violence.[67] Gandhi stated; "Live simply so that others might simply live."[68] Socrates in Plato's republic advocates a vegetarian diet for greater peace and health in mankind. He predicted not only ill health, but a greater likelihood of war in a society that consumes meat.[69] Do we in fact nourish ourselves on the fear of the animals we so violently slaughter in terror? Do we put ourselves into a type of karmic debt? I believe that what goes around comes around, do good and good will come to you.

We've already lost 75% of our top soil.[70] The growing demands we're putting on our land is leading us into certain destruction. Eighty five percent of the top soil loss of our land is directly related to livestock production.[71] Furthermore, the more we erode our soil the more dependent on others we become for our food. As a result of so much soil erosion and top soil depletion we act by clearing new land to replace it. We also pave this land for urbanization purposes. Now for each acre we use for urbanization, 7 acres are used for livestock production.[72] At this rate forests in the United States will be gone in only 50 years.[73] Without trees and or a with reduction in them, our climate is drastically affected. This will lead to flooding, a loss of plants and animals, an inability to naturally purify our water, and finally the loss of the wonderful beauty and resulting inspiration nature affords us. In looking at the destruction of the tropical rain forests in Central and South America, at the current rate of deforestation, they should be entirely gone in about 40 years.[74] This is a devastating thought knowing that they contain 80% of the earth's vegetation and 50% of all the wild living species of the world.[75] The rate of destruction is at about 1000 species a year.[76] In the next thirty years at this rate of destruction, over a million species will become extinct, most of the world's oxygen supply, and a quarter of our medicines will be mere history.

Another primary resource of concern is our water supply. In the United States over 50% of our water supply is used for livestock production.[77] To add insult to injury enormous amounts of water are necessary for excrement removal alone. It takes 2500 gallons of water to process 11 lbs. of meat.[78] Four thousand gallons of water is necessary to support a meat eater's diet for one day, as opposed to only 300 gallons to support a vegan's.[79] Another amazing fact is that the water necessary to process (raise, slaughter, etc.) a 1000 lb. steer would be sufficient to float a destroyer ship.[80] The costs and depletion of our water supply is a serious economic and ecological problem. As a result of the scarcity of water as a resource, we need to seek alternate modes of generating electricity. To better illustrate the exorbitant costs of water depletion to us, if the California water supply for livestock raising was discontinued, the income that could be added to other businesses would be over ten billion dollars a year.[81]

Putting aside the massive costs to us that come from water usage in livestock production we can add to the atrocity knowing the correlation between environmental pollution and this industry. As little as fifty or so years ago animal wastes were returned to the soil. Today in an era of factory organized production, there's two very negative side effects. Besides the excessive stripping of topsoil and soil erosion we have to concern ourselves with where the chemical fertilizers, pesticides, and wastes from the animals end up in terms of the environment. Much of these wastes end up in our private and public water supplies.[82] These wastes, high in nitrogen, if not put back into the soil turn into ammonia and nitrates.[83] These compounds are linked to serious brain damage in infants.[84] Wastes from meat processing of itself contributes to our country's hazardous water pollution more than 3x's as much as all other industries together. Over a billion tons of waste a year is linked to livestock production.[85]

Yes, there's hardly enough justification for a meat based diet when we know that in the production of livestock we use one third of the raw materials used for any purposes.[86] In further support of a vegan diet is knowing that soybeans are 40 times more efficient as fuel for our bodies than meat.[87] Our bodies get much more energy per available calories from soybeans.

Yes, because all things are connected in nature, our very choices of food have a tremendous effect on our survival, our children's survival, the survival of other species, and the overall survival of our planet. Isn't it strange to be paying such a high price for our destruction, when we can pay so much less for our survival?

In Ecclesiastes 3:19 of the bible, there is also a reference to how our fate is that of the animals around us. "For that which befalleth the sons of men befalleth the beasts. Even one thing befalleth them: as the one dieth, so dieth the other; yea, they have all one breath, so that a man hath no preeminence above a beast."

Our American ideals of competition and money at all costs contribute to the sacrificing of our health, sanity, and the welfare of others. Throughout my life I strove to be different figuring that which was common wasn't special or precious. It was a natural inclination for me to choose vegetarianism. By the time I had done enough reading to logically substantiate such a choice I was thoroughly convinced I'd made the right decision. Ironically, if the majority of Americans were vegetarians, I would of probably been seeking another alternative.

As a natural innovator I'd like to go a step further to illustrate the need for an extreme turn in our directions. I'll question whether the diet of the horse is an even closer model of perfection. Looking at this creature of grace, strength, endurance and beauty, what could possibly be the harm and not the good of seeking it as a model for one's self. By looking at a horse's diet, we can see clearly that its absolutely a pure vegetarian one. First of all horses consume between 6 and 8 gallons of water a day. The majority of their diet consists of hay from wheat, alfalfa, barley and soybeans. This would compose about 75% of their diet. About 20% of their diet is composed of cubes made from various combinations of corn, soybeans, oats, Brewer's yeast, molasses, vitamins (especially A & D), calcium supplements, limestone and other trace minerals. The remaining 5% of their diet is in fibrous foods including wheat bran, whey and linseed meal. Linseed oil is often added to a horse's diet to improve their coats and add luster. Other foods consumed by horses in small quantities periodically are: peas, rice, carrots, apples, beets, potatoes, turnips, honey, molasses and sugar.

I personally have easily sustained myself on a healthy diet of oatmeal, tofu, whole wheat bread, vegetable stews, peas, beans, corn, potatoes, carrot juice, fruit, and alfalfa supplements. The only thing I might additionally add to satisfy my more human cravings is some spaghetti sauce for my tofu sandwiches. For liquids I use rice milk, apple juice, and water. So really how far fetched is a horse's diet from our own? My own weight is hardly a problem. My digestion and energy levels are the best I've known. In addition I rarely fall victim to eating when I'm not really hungry but just seeking carnal pleasure. The cost of such a diet on my pocketbook, my health, and the health of the planet is minimal. I also find, I never struggle to look in shape or keep extra lbs. off, which wasn't always the case. As a result of the low fat, salt and sugar content of it, I don't store a lot of excess calories. The food I consume is easily broken down by my body, not prone to lay dormant as toxins inside of me. Vegetables have the lowest level of pesticides on them of all foods. Finally, I nourish myself better than most people, without inflicting unnecessary suffering on the other living creatures I share the planet with. I live with a lighter conscious and a better karma.

In "The Complete Horsebook" the author states: " The nutrients required to keep a horse in good health are not unlike those of humans."[88] Horses as humans, when compared to cows, have smaller stomachs and a larger intestinal tract for digestion. Hence, bulk and fiber are important for us to feel satiated and to help food pass through the long winding canals of our intestines. In comparison, carnivores have a relatively short intestinal tract especially in the colon, which doesn't allow the putrefaction of toxins, so likely to occur in our intestines, where food tends to linger. Meat and dairy products tend towards toxicity more so than fruits, vegetables and grains.

There exist a small percentage of people who hold tirelessly to their ideals and convictions. Mahatma Gandhi and Isadora Duncan were amongst the great ones. Gandhi was a man thoroughly bound to his convictions. One of Gandhi's strongest convictions was that of upholding to nonviolence. He adhered to this ideal in his pursuit of world peace as in his own existence. He demonstrated stringent self-discipline in all aspects of his existence, in order to uphold what he considered to be the purest of morals in his behavior. This was inherent in but not exclusive to his commitment towards vegetarianism. He was known to nearly starve rather than relinquish himself to what he considered any less pure a diet. He adhered to eating very bland food often professing; "The real seat of taste was not the tongue but the mind…."[89]

Violence is subtly bred in us as we grow up in our culture. Fathers often encourage fishing and hunting for sport, not as a necessity for food as was once the case. Parents encourage their kids to not be bullied in school. When their son might brag about "beating the crap out of so and so," it's often condoned if not commended. Children attending public schools carry guns, knives, and other weapons to either offend or defend themselves. The prevalence of a machismo attitude is not necessarily an ugly manner, but it carries the principles of violence with it.

Drug use and the need to obtain more money in the quickest and easiest manner, regardless of the ugliness and karma attached to it, has allowed organized crime to inundate our society with violence and modes of abuse towards each other. Violence and a lack of integrity laces all aspects of our society. Unscrupulous doctors and lawyers thrive on the misery of others more often than might be believed. Continuing to keep hopelessly ill people alive in order to profit from the medical insurance money, has forced us to focus on the issue of euthanasia.

Only through a higher consciousness that is willing to question the integrity of all our actions, can we better ourselves and the world we live in. It's only our ignorance, callousness and greediness, that could encourage us to close our eyes to a more noble avenue of existence. Where will it all lead us, all these mounting lifestyle sins we're accumulating? Not only to our own painful ends, but to the ends of those around us, and preceding us... Start by caring, you do make a difference!

CHAPTER SIX

Is Utopia an Absurd Vision?

The direction you choose in health and fitness for yourself, will influence the direction of the planet.

As far back as the ancient Greek and Romans, man at times considered a holistic approach to health and fitness. We are beginning to evolve from a piece meal approach of more recent past generations, to a more holistic one as we enter the 21st century. We are considering more than just the appearance of ourselves and the things around us as we consider the content. We could look great on the surface, but may be diseased internally. Our environment might look beautiful, but in its hull it may harbor the most toxic of elements to life. As we peel away the skin of our environment and selves, we'll see and understand more fully that to really get the full benefits of life, we need to search deeper and work harder than we may have once realized. We the people of the 21th century want more; the expectations of what we want out of life correlates with our growing base of information.

Since nature is perfect, it will reward us for living in harmony with its laws. By living by its laws we prosper. The greatest biological relationship under the laws of nature is mutualism; and in order to achieve this relationship with nature we have much work to do. After all, for so many centuries, so many of us have had a parasitic relationship with her. Just as in most of these types of relationships the host eventually dies or is destroyed. Unfortunately, if the host dies in the case of nature being the host, there are no more hosts for the parasites (us) to turn to and so we too vanish.

It is my belief that through Humanism, self-expression, and in being informed, we can obtain and exercise those ideals that will enable us to achieve a higher consciousness and superior human attributes. The offspring of this achievement in oneself is to better facilitate global harmony and prosperity. After all, these benefits begin with ourselves, within our minds (education), within the food we eat (diet), and within our bodies. Less toxic bodies means a less toxic planet. Our offspring will be healthier, our excrement less toxic, and a less toxic atmosphere will prevail.

A collective superior state of consciousness isn't possible until enough individuals achieve it.

How could we ever expect to realize a dream like world peace, when we're at war with ourselves? Yes indeed, peace begins at home in all our kitchens and all our hearts. There are many pathways to a more peaceful, kinder, and healthier heart. These include: self-expression, self-security and reduced jealousy. Self-security is derived through self-knowledge and is a result of sufficient self-expression. Prancercise® is one vehicle towards nurturing one's self-expression; the side benefits are physical prosperity and fitness.

Wouldn't it be a real blessing if what we ate, thought and did for the improvement of our physical appearance also benefited others and the planet? Why do we limit our interest to me, me,me? Even in a man/woman relationship this can't work. Why do we take it further into nature?

Dr. Leo Buscaglia professes that the most important subject of all in the world is that of love. There wasn't even a class in love offered to students in our schools, until he initiated one within the last two decades. We're all mirror images of each other (reflections), and if we don't like ourselves we can't really like others. If we downright hate ourselves we can more readily hate others. What if, we could condition ourselves to have more self-love each day by doing simple things that we know are good for us, and we enjoy? If we look forward to doing these things and therefore wish to continue them, and if each time we do them we're rewarded, and those all around us are too, how could we not be thrilled at the thought of this? Wellness is contagious and can become a very strong habit. If we had a choice of addictions soon after we were born (pure of ideas and influence), do you suspect we'd choose self-destructive ones? It's unlikely we'd choose this fate which is but an exercise in negative conditioning, basically learned and acquired from the people of influence around us. These influences prevail before we've even learned basic logic and judgment to ward against them. It's more likely that our instinctive drives would be ones that were in line with our survival. Man, who has turned away and strayed from his instincts due to civilizing influences has created a troublesome dilemma. If man relies on his thought process, by which he can justify most anything to himself, more than he relies on his instincts, he could easily lead himself into destruction. Another tendency man has is his need to be led, to follow. So if many men follow a few men with warped thought processes then the masses will eventually meet their destruction. Learning to think for yourself and make your own decisions is not the American way. If you wish to do so you'll probably find yourself fighting all kinds of accepted standards and practices. However, if you realize how very vital this fight is for your survival, and that of the planet's, you should be less inclined to hesitate in doing so. Is looking and doing our best not beyond make up, clothes, P.T.A. meetings, pledging to charities, going to church or temple? Isn't this just the surface that doesn't really get to the crux of what's doing and being our best? Consider ancient Greece or Rome, where a man who was as knowledgeable in art, music, literature, logic and philosophy, as he was developed in physical fitness and self-defense, was considered a superior human being. Why then are we so many hundreds of years later so piece meal in our approach to our own self-development? Are we conditioning our bodies towards flexibility and quickness, or merely strength and power? Our minds and way of thinking relate to and reflect the types of bodies we contain. If our bodies are flexible and quick, so too our minds can follow… Synchronization of both in order to achieve the most harmonious survival mode should be our quests.

I contain a Utopian vision of how a more just and loving society would be. First of all, this society would be governed by nonviolence, with full respect for human life. All resources would be shared so that everyone would be provided for. Additional resources would be granted to those who provided additional services, beyond what was required for securing a maintenance level. Criminals would be isolated and forced to live entirely with each other on an island or in a separate contained city. Victimless crimes would no longer be criminal. Marriage would be non-contractual. In a man/woman relationship commitment would be verbal, and if dissolved the men would go before a judge to assure proper care for the women and children. There would be no need for court intervention as long as the women and children were self-sufficient or being assisted by the estranged man. This would eliminate expense and the temptation of trying to get more than they needed. There would exist community child care, and other similar services, where those volunteers that offer their services are rewarded with additional resources. Education would be treated in the same fashion as would public works. There would be no need for taxation because all necessities would be covered by volunteers who would be trained individuals, compensated for their additional services. Besides, there would be no real income. Schools of the arts would flourish where children could be encouraged at an early age to develop modes of self-expression. School would only be required at an elementary level, above this would be optional. Independent study would be encouraged as an option, knowing requirements would need to be met to receive adult privileges later such as driving and career choices for further education. Hence, if society was founded upon the principles of love, desire, individual expression, and mutually beneficial relationships that were win win, the world could be a remarkably different and a beautiful place to live in. People would live by guiding their behavior to consider not only their own betterment, but the betterment of everyone. Where everyone shared cooperatively, and the few didn't benefit at the cost of many... where children were encouraged to be individuals not carbon copy citizens. This way, uniquely gifted individuals might find their special purpose in life at an early age, within the delicate web of society. Certainly by crippling them with the standard avenues of required education up until 18 years of age, this potential achievement is less likely to materialize. Is it any wonder that so many individuals are so rebellious today, especially our youth? So much protesting, so many destructive addictions (self-destruction), so much violence (destruction of others), so much discontent in general... You might say to yourself we'll never have those conditions that will please everyone; this is surely true…however, there would have to be some improvement over the ocean of discontent that exists today.

The American society is one of the greatest societies currently known to man. This is a shallow statement, however, we have leaps and bounds to go in order to have a society based on love of our fellow man instead of greed. Instead of millions of dollars being spent on plastic surgery, why aren't we aiding the less privileged? Almost every Thanksgiving I was going to the hospital to visit some sorry souls that are alone for the holiday. My father died of a sudden heart attack on Thanksgiving eve and spent it in the hospital. Who are we to shuffle through our middle class palaces to partake in a feast fit for a king? We are so removed from the less privileged, how could we really feel deep in our souls, how really fortunate we are? How could we feel so when most of us deny contributions or aid to the less privileged? Many of us are poorly conditioned hypocrites that find it easier to follow each other into empty dark spaces than consider another path for ourselves.

One must be able to envision a better way of living before they're able to work toward one. Unless you take the time and have the nature to question things as they are, and perceive beyond our very noses, how can we expect people to desire better? We all are very special human beings in our own ways, so I plead to you don't bury yourself in booze, drugs gambling, sex, education, fitness, music or anything else so much that you become numb to what's happening beyond your small worlds. I suspect many of us bury ourselves in destructive or even somewhat constructive obsessions, because we're partially aware of our greater purpose in life, and feel helpless towards doing something about it. Let's not numb our consciences to what we know in our hearts is right, instead, let's face what's right head on, and resist what we know is wrong.

Yes, this book was meant to help direct you towards a more meaningful life, partly through exercise and unique physical expression, partly through your unique mental expression, and partly through illustrating the need there is to consider more than our own individual welfare, in order to have our individual welfare.

ENDNOTES

Chapter One

1 Podhajsky, Alois, Complete Training of Horse and Rider, In the Principles of Classical Horsemanship, trans., Podhajsky, Eva and Williams, V.D.S., Colonel, (New York: Doubleday and Co. Inc., 1967), p.17

2 Ibid

3 Duncan, Irma, Duncan Dancer, (New York: Books for Libraries, a division of Arno Press, 1980), p.211

4 Jowitt, Deborah, Time and the Dancing Image, (New York: Wm. Morrow and Co Inc., 1988), taken from: Euripides, The Bacchae

5 Goodman, Linda, Linda Goodman's Sun Signs, (New York: Bantam Books, 1968), p.126

6 Gutlin, Bernard, "Effect of Increases in physical and mental stress, Research Quarterly, 37:211, May, 1966

7 Hart, Marcia, E. and Shay, Clayton, J., "Relationship between Physical Fitness and Academic Success," Research Quarterly, 35:445, Oct. 1964

8 Health Maintenance through Physical Conditioning, ed., Cantu, Robert, M.D., (Mass.: PSG Publishing Co. Inc., 1981) pp.14 22

9 Ibid

10 Ibid

11 Ibid

12 Strauss, Sally, Inner Rhythm, An Exciting Approach to Stress Free Living, (San Francisco: Chase Publications, 1984), p.44

Chapter Two

1 Sorell, Walter, The Dancer's Image, Points and Counterpoints, (New York: Columbia University Press, 1971), p.9

2 Ibid, p.19

3 Ibid, p.79

4 Ibid, p.170.

5 Ibid, p.171

6   Ibid, p.188
7   Ibid, p.190
8   Ibid, p.373
9   Ibid
10 Ibid, p.303
11 Ibid, p.396
12 Ibid
13 Ibid, p.397
14 Ibid
15 Ibid, p.410
16 Ibid, p.414
17 Ibid, p.441
18 As per note 3, Duncan, p.127
19 Ibid. pp.83 84
20 Ibid
21 Ibid
22 Schneider, Ilyich, Ilya, Isadora Duncan: The Russian Years, (New York: Harcourt Brace and World Inc., 1968), p.39
23 As per note 3, Duncan, p.25
24 Ibid
25 Ibid
26 Blair, Fredrika, Isadora: Portrait of the Artist as a Woman, (New York: McGraw Hill Book Co., 1986), p.67
27 Ibid, p.23
28 Ibid, p.29
29 Ibid, p.44
30 Ibid, p.60
31 Ibid
32 Ibid, p.240
33 Ibid, p.275, taken from a quote by Paris Singer in: Stokes, Sewell, Isadora, An Intimate Portrait (London: Bretano, 1928), p. 152
34 As per note 24, Blair, p.288
35 Ibid, p.387
36 Ibid, p.392, taken from: Desti, Mary, The Untold Story, (New York: N.P.), 1929.
37 As per note 24, p.396
38 Ibid

39 Ibid, p.400
40 Ibid
41 Jowitt, Deborah, Time and the Dancing Image, p.80
42 As per note 1, Sorell, p.373
43 As per note 39, Jowitt, p. 90.
44 As per note 24, Blair, p. 405
45 Ibid, p.407
46 Concerning the Spiritual in Art, trans., Sadler, M.T., (New York: Dover Publications Inc., 1977), p.90

Chapter Three

1 Sorell, Walter, The Dancer's Image, Points and Counterpoints, p.74
2 Ibid, p.73
3 Ibid, p.76
4 Ibid, p.151
5 Epictetus, Discourses and Enchiridion, trans., Higginson, Wentworth, Thomas, (New York: Walter J. Black, 1944), p.119
6 Ibid, p.122
7 Aristotle, On Man in the Universe, ed., Loomis, Louis, (New York: Walter J. Black, 1943), p.99
8 Ibid, p.87
9 Aurelius, Marcus, Marcus Aurelius, and his Times, (New York: Walter J. Black, 1945), pp.21 22
10 Ibid, p.27
11 Plato, trans., Jowett, B., ed. Loomis, Rope, Louise, (New York: Walter J Black, 1942), p.288
12 Ibid, p.289
13 Strauss, Sally, Inner Rhythm, p.44
14 Ibid, p.51; also: Halpern, Steven, Sound Health, the Music that Makes Us Whole (New York: Harper and Row Inc., 1985), p.61.
15 Snyder, Paul, Health and Human Nature, (Penn.: Chilton Book Co., 1980), p.69
16 Ibid, p.148
17 The Essential Gandhi, His Life, Work and Ideas, An Anthology, ed. Fischer, Louis, (New York: Vintage Books, 1962), p.35

18 Fischer, Louis, The Life of Mahatma Gandhi, (New York: Harper and Row, 1950), p.329

19 Ibid, p.166

20 Strauss, Sally, Inner Rhythm, p.51

Chapter Four

1 Chaffee, Ellen and Greisheimer, Esther, Basic Anatomy and Physiology, (Philadelphia: J.B. Lippincott co., 1969), pp.112 186

2 Jacob, Ellen, Dancing, A Guide for the Dancer You Can Be, (N.P.: Addison Wesley Publishing Co., 1981), p.227

3 Berardi, GiGi, Finding Balance, Fitness Training for a Lifetime in Dance, (Princeton: Dance Horizons Book Co., 1991), pp.58 60

4 Ibid, p.80.

5 Ibid, pp.97 151

6 As per note 2, Jacob, pp.236 250

Chapter Five

1 Robbins, John, Diet for A New America, (New Hamp.: Stillpoint Publishing, 1987), p.380

2 Ibid, p.37

3 Ibid, p.41, taken from: Fox, M., Returning to Eden, (N.P.: Viking Press, 1980), pp.10 11

4 As per note 1, p.38

5 Ibid, p.53. 6   Ibid, p.54

7 Ibid, p.55

8 Ibid, p.56

9 Ibid, p.57, taken from: Angstom, C.I., " Mechanical Failures Plague Cage Layers," Onondaga County Farm News, Dec. 1970, p.13

10 As per note 1, p.58, taken from H. Reed as a personal communication to John Robbins of Diet for A New America

11 As per note 1, p.59

12 Ibid, p.61

13 Ibid, p.63, taken from: " Scientist Studies Test Tube Pig," Hog Farm Management, April, 1975, p.61

14 As per note 1, p. 64, taken from: Mason, J and Singer, P., Animal Factories, (N.P.: Crown Publishers, 1980), p.42

15 Ibid, taken from: Gowe, R.S., Director of the Animal Research Institute, Agriculture Canada, at the conference on "Livestock Intensive Methods of Production," OTTAWA, Dec. 6 7, 1978

16 As per note 1, pp.65 66, taken from: Mason, J. and Singer P., Animal Factories, pp.56 58

17 Ibid, Animal Factories, p.29.

18 As per note 1, p. 67, taken from: Shurter, D. and Walter, E., " The Meat You Eat," The Plain Truth, Oct. Nov., 1970

19 As per note 1, p. 74

20 Ibid, p.80

21 Ibid, p.81, taken from: Schell, O., Modern Meat, (N.P.: Vantage Books, 1985), PP;61 62

22 As per note 1, p.84, taken from: Animal Factories, p.30

23 As per note 1, p.85, taken from: Farm Farm Journal, April, 1970

24 As per note 1, p.85

25 Ibid, p.86

26 Ibid, p.87, taken from: Animal Factories

27 As per note 1, p.89, taken from: Singer, P., Animal Liberation, (N.P.: Avon Books, 1975), p.114

28 As per note 1, p.90

29 As per note 1, p.93, taken from: Animal Factories, p.63

30 Ibid, p.93

31 As per note 1, p.94, taken from: " Pig Health Loses Total $187 Million," Farm Journal, Sept. 1978, p. Hog 2

32 As per note 1, pp.95 96

33 Ibid, p.105

34 Ibid, taken from: Brynes, J., "Raising Pigs by the Calendar at Maplewood Farm," Hog Farm Management, Sept. 1976, p.30

35 As per note 1, p.105

36 Ibid, p.107

37 Ibid, taken from: Handbook of Livestock Management Techniques, (N.P.: Burgess Publishers, 1981)

38 As per note 1, p.110, taken from:
    a) Giehl, D., Vegetarianism, (N.P.: Harper and Row, 1979), pp.119 120

b) Hightower, J.,Eat Your Heart Out, (N.P.: Crown Publishers, 1975), p.99

c) Hunter, B., Consumer Beware, (N.P.: Simon and Schuster, 1971),pp.113 114

d) Lappe, M.F., Diet For A Small Planet, (N.P.: Ballantine, 1982), pp.67 68

e) Schell, O., Modern Meat, (N.P.: Vintage Books, 1985), pp. 125 126, 137,143, 148 149, 167, 179 180. f) Singer, P., Animal Liberation, p.129

g) Singer, P., and Mason, J., Animal Factories, pp. 29 30, 48 49, 72

h) Sussman, V., The Vegetarian Alternative, (N.P.: Rodale Press, 1978), pp.173 174

39 As per note 1, p.111

40 Ibid

41 Ibid, p.112

42 Ibid, p.113

44 Ibid, p.116

45 Ibid, p.117

46 As per note 1, pp. 140 141, taken from: Singer, P., Animal Liberation, p.153

47 As per note 1, p.171

48 As per note 1, p.155, taken from: Hur, Robin, Food Reform: Our Desperate Need,

(N.P.: Heidleberg Publishers, 1975), p.95

49 As per note 1, p.154, taken from: Kapleau, Philip, (San Francisco: Harper and Row, 1981), p.67

50 As per note 1, p.157, taken from: Fisher, Irving, " The Influence of Flesh Eating on Endurance," Yale Medical Journal, 1907, 13(5): 205 221

51 As per note 1, p.158

52 Ibid, p.163

53 As per note 1, p.173, taken from: Scrimshaw, N., "An Analysis of Past and Present Recommended Dietary Allowances for Protein in Health and Disease," The New England Journal of Medicine, Jan. 22, 1976, p.200

54 As per note 1, pp.189 190

55 Ibid, p.253

56 Ibid, pp.266 267

57 Ibid, p.275

58 Ibid, p.303

59 Ibid, p.312 313

60 Ibid, p.314

61 As per note 1, p.331, taken from: Regenstein, L., How To Survive In America The Poisoned, (N.P.: Acropolis Books, 1982), p.298

62 As per note 1, p.345, taken from: Boyle, R., and Environmental Defense Fund, (N.P.: Alfred Knopf, 1979), pp.206 207; and: A Brief Review of Selected Environmental Contamination Incidents with a Potential for Health Effects," prepared by the Library of Congress, for the Committee on Environment and Public Works, U.S. Senate, Aug.1980, p.289

63 As per note 1, pp.350 355, taken from: "The Food Crisis: the Shortages May Pit the `Have Nots' against the ` Haves, ' The Wall Street Journal, Oct. 3, 1974, p.20

64 As per note 1, p.351, taken from: Lappe, Moore, Francis, Diet For A Small Planet, Tenth Anniversary ed., (New York: Ballantine Books, 1982), p.69

65 As per note 1, p.351

66 Ibid, p.353

67 Ibid, p.354

68 Ibid, p.355

69 Plato, trans., B. Jowett, ed., Louise Loomis, (New York: Walter J. Black), 1942

70 As per note 1, p.357, taken from: " Six Inches From Starvation, How and Why America's Topsoil is Disappearing," Vegetarian Times, March 1985, pp. 45 47. 71   As per note 1, p.358, taken from:

a) Diet For A Small Planet, quote from Robin Hur, p.80

b) Land Degradation: " Effects on Food and Energy Resources," Pimental, et al, Science, vol. 194, Oct. 1976

c) "Soil and Water Resources Conservation Act Summary of Appraisal," U.S.D.A. Review Draft, 1980, p.18

d) "Soil Degradation:" Effects on Agricultural Productivity," by the National Association of Conservation Districts, W.D.C., Interim

    Report Number Four, National Agricultural Lands Study, 1980, p.20

e) National Resource Capital in U.S. Agriculture: Irrigation, Drainage and Conservation Investments Since 1900, E.S.C.S. Staff Paper, March, 1979

72 As per note 1, taken from: Hur, Robin and Fields, David, "Are High Fat Diets Killing Our Forests?" Vegetarian Times, Feb. 1984

73 As per note 1, p.362

74 As per note 1, p.363. 75   Ibid, pp.363 364

76 As per note 1, p.365, taken from: " Acres U.S.A.," Kansas City, Missouri, vol. 15, no. 6, June, 1985, p.2

77 As per note 1, p.367, taken from: Diet For A Small Planet, p.69

78 As per note 1, p.367, taken from: Borgstrom, Georg, "Presentation to the Annual Meeting of the American Association for the Advancement of Science," 1981

79 As per note 1, p.367, taken from: Altschul, Aaron, " Proteins Their Chemistry and Politics," (N.P.: Basic Books, 1965), p.264

80 As per note 1, p.367, taken from: "The Browning of America," Newsweek, Feb. 22, 1981, p.26

81 As per note 1, p.370, taken from: Hur, Robin, and Fiels, David, "America's Appetite for Meat is Ruining Our Water," Vegetarian Times, Jan. 1985

82 As per note 1, p.372

83 Ibid

84 As per note1, p.373. 85   Ibid, taken from: Lappe, Moore, Francis, Diet For A Small Planet, 1975 ed., cited from Georg Borgstrum, p.22

86 As per note 1, p.374

87 As per note 1, p.376, taken from: Pimental, David, " Energy and Land Constraints in Food Protein Production," Science, Nov. 21, 1975

88 The Complete Horsebook, ed., Elwyn Hartley Edward, and Canida Geddes, (Vermont: Trafalger Square Inc., 1988), p.188

89 The Essential Gandhi His Life, Work and Work and Ideas, An Anthology, ed., Louis Fischer, (New York: Vintage Books, 1962), p.26

ABOUT THE AUTHOR:

Joanna Rohrback graduated Westchester Community College with an Associates in Science degree, after which she attended The University of Miami School of Nursing and went on to graduate with honors, from Florida Atlantic University with a Bachelor's degree in Health Services.

She worked as a Social Worker for the State of Florida for several years and then as a Realtor. She created her Prancercise®Program in 1989 as well as the video Funky Punky's Prancercise Program. Shortly thereafter she founded the Vegetarian Advocate's Group. She finished and copyrighted her book <u>Prancercise®:The Art of Physical and Spiritual</u> <u>Excellence</u> as an unpublished manuscript in 1994. Joanna later went on to facilitate a Food Addictions Support group for several years and organized the Citizen's for Democracy Group. Joanna was a full-time caretaker for her mother during which time she did research for Jennifer Van Bergen, a journalist. Joanna had her own article published "Model to Monstrosity:The Emergency Health Powers Act" in the SunCoast Eco Report (Feb./March 2003) also online at: http://www.iahf.com/20030117.html and an editorial in New Times April 17-23 2003.

Joanna donates time consulting the Elderly and Disabled on the benefits of holistic medicine and supports environmental issues facing her community; she is currently owner/manager of Prancercise®, L.L.C., and www.Prancercise.com, through which she teaches her aerobics and does Wellness Coaching.